the fussy baby book

Also by the same authors:

The Baby Book
The Good Behaviour Book
The Baby Sleep Book

the fussy baby book

Parenting your high-need child
from birth to age five

Dr William Sears and Martha Sears, R.N.

Edited by Caroline Deacon

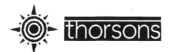

Thorsons
An Imprint of HarperCollins*Publishers*
77–85 Fulham Palace Road,
Hammersmith, London W6 8JB

The website address is: www.thorsonselement.com

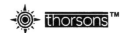

and *Thorsons* are trademarks of
HarperCollins*Publishers* Ltd

First published in the USA in 1996 by Little, Brown and Company

This revised and updated edition published in 2005 by Thorsons

A catalogue record of this book
is available from the British Library

ISBN 978-0-00-733214-4

contents

II: the high-need child grows up 165

III: stories from the experts 225

acknowledgements

Much of the material in this book comes from our on-the-job parenting of our own high-need children. Besides our personal stories, we have included ideas that many parents of high-need children have sent us. A special thanks to Kathy Nesper for her story of the high-need thrill ride in Chapter 11; Gina Baker-Basler for her review of the manuscript and for contributing advice on mother burnout in Chapter 7; Georgianna Rodiger, Ph.D., for her insight and critique of the manuscript; and the hundreds of mothers and fathers who have contributed their advice and stories, especially Gwen Gotsch, Tina Henningson, and McCall Gordon. We thank Tracee Zeni for her untiring assistance in the typing and preparation of the manuscript. We are particularly grateful to our editor, Jennifer Josephy, and our copyeditor, Pamela Marshall, for their patience and help in our many rewrites. Finally, we thank our own children, who taught us the art of listening to their needs.

a word from
dr bill and martha

We want to both congratulate and encourage you on being blessed with a high-need child. Having a challenging child will bring out the best and worst in you; we wish to help this life-changing experience bring out the best.

Parenting a high-need child is like attending a continuous life-enrichment seminar. From the moment these infants exit the womb, in one way or another, they announce, "Hi, Mum and Dad. You've been blessed with an above-average child, and I need above-average parenting. If you give it to me, we're going to get along fine; but if you don't, we're going to have a bit of trouble down the road." And these babies have the persistence required to hold up their end of this bargain. Right from the start these children make it clear they need *more!* The good news is they also give more to everyone who cares for them.

This book is about children who are challenging and the parents who guide them. Besides insights that we have gained from parenting our own high-need children and from counselling hundreds of parents in our paediatric practice, sprinkled throughout this book you will find testimonies from parents who have survived and thrived with their high-need children – kids you would like. We let the experts speak for themselves.

Parenting a high-need child will be one of the most difficult journeys of your life. It will also be one of the most rewarding.

William and Martha Sears
San Clemente, California
May 1996

I

the journey begins

Parenting is a journey. Parenting a high-need child is a journey where you unwittingly end up in uncharted territory. Before your baby's birth you imagine what the journey will be like. You buy guidebooks. You listen to friends who have taken similar trips. It's exciting. Your baby is born and the journey begins. Suddenly your trip isn't going as planned. Your child is not following the guidebooks. He takes you on a different journey, one that you might not have chosen and certainly not the one you had anticipated. Initially, you resent this change in travel plans. The road is bumpy. It is lonely. And it's costing you much more energy than you had budgeted. But you've purchased a non-refundable ticket, so you must go on. While your friends are seeing all the popular sights, your child pulls you off the usual paths, down side roads, and into places where you're forced to carve some new trails on your own. The trip is tiring and challenging. You have difficulty sharing your discoveries with your friends; they haven't been where you've been or seen the world through your child's eyes. Before long, though, you will gradually begin to realize how much richer your life is and how much wiser you are for having experienced this special journey.

chapter 1

hayden – our high-need child

Sitting in the high school auditorium one spring evening, we proudly watched our seventeen-year-old daughter, Hayden, take her bows following the school's production of *Oklahoma!* She'd played the role of Ado Annie wonderfully, yet it was the Hayden we saw after the curtain call who warmed our hearts the most.

We watched how she cared for her friends – the eye contact, the hugs, the delightfully natural social gestures, and the expressivity that drew people, magnet-like, into her presence. As a tear or two flowed down her dad's cheeks, we thought back to "Hayden the handful" – the demanding baby, the strong-minded toddler, the challenging preschooler, the full-of-energy grade-schooler, and the exhausting teen. Now we are seeing a dynamic adult beginning to emerge. How the three of us got through those years and to this point in our lives inspired this book. Here's the story of the baby we got and the lessons we learned.

how she acted

Hayden stretched us as parents and as individuals. Our first three children were relatively "easy" infants. They slept well and had a predictable feeding routine. Their needs were easy to identify – and satisfy. In fact, I began to suspect that parents in my paediatric practice who complained about their fussy babies were exaggerating. "What's all the fuss about difficult babies?" I wondered.

Then came Hayden, our fourth, whose birth changed our lives. Our first clue that she was going to be different came within a day or two. "I can't put her down", became Martha's recurrent theme. Breast-feeding for Hayden was not only a source of food, but also a constant source of comfort. Martha became a human pacifier.

Hayden would not accept substitutes. She was constantly in arms and at her mother's breast – and after a while those arms and breasts would get tired. Hayden's cries were not mere complaints, they were all-out alarms. Well-meaning friends suggested, "Just put her down and let her cry it out." That didn't work at all. Her extraordinary persistence kept her crying. Her cries did not fade away. They intensified if we didn't respond.

Hayden was very good at teaching us what she needed. "As long as we hold her, she's content" became our baby-care slogan. If we tried letting her fuss, she only fussed harder. We played "pass the baby". When Martha's arms gave out, into mine Hayden came. We used a front-pack carrier we had saved from brother Peter's baby days, but Hayden liked it only when we were out walking.

Nights were not bad in the early months, considering how intense she was by day. But around six months that all changed, and her nights became high-need. She rejected her cot as if it were a cage. After fourteen hours of baby holding, we longed for some nighttime relief. Hayden had other plans. As soon as we put her down in her cot and tried to creep out of the bedroom, she would awaken, howling in protest at having been left alone. Martha would nurse her back to sleep in the rocking chair, then put her back into her cot, and after an hour or less she would awaken again, demanding a repeat of the rocking-chair-and-nursing routine. It soon became evident that Hayden's need for human contact was as high at night as it was during the day.

how we felt

If Hayden had been our first child, we would have concluded that it was our fault she couldn't settle herself, since we were inexperienced parents. But she was our fourth child, and by this time we felt we had a handle on caring for children. Nevertheless, Hayden did cause us to doubt our parenting abilities. Our confidence was getting shaky as our energy reserves were nearing empty. Our feelings about Hayden were as erratic as her behaviour. Some days we were empathetic and nurturing; other days we were exhausted, confused, and resentful of her constant demands. Such mixed feelings were foreign to us, especially after parenting three easily managed babies. Soon it became obvious that Hayden was a different kind of baby. She was wired differently from other babies.

lesson

It wasn't our fault. Hayden fussed because of her temperament, not because of our parenting abilities.

The challenge for us was to figure out how to mother and father this unique little person while also conserving enough energy for our other three children – and ourselves.

Our first obstacle to overcome was our professional past. We were educated in the fifties and sixties, so we were victims of the prevailing parenting mind-set of those times – fear of spoiling. We entered parenthood believing it was mandatory to control our children lest they control us. And there was that horrible fear of being manipulated. Were we losing control? Was Hayden manipulating us? We consulted books, a useless exercise. No baby book contained a chapter on Hayden. And the mostly male authors were either beyond child-rearing age or seemed far removed from the trenches of everyday baby tending. Yet here we were, two experienced adults, whose lives were being taken over by a ten-pound infant.

Hayden opened us up as people. The turning point came when we closed the baby books and opened our hearts to our child. Instead of defensively getting caught up in the fear of spoiling, we started listening to what Hayden had been trying to tell us from the moment she exited the womb. As soon as we discarded our preconceived ideas of how babies are supposed to be and accepted the reality of how Hayden was, we all got along much better.

If she fussed when we put her down but was content when we held her, we would hold her. If she needed to feed a lot, Martha would feed her. We believed Hayden knew what she needed, and fortunately she had the persistence to keep telling us until we understood.

lesson

Hayden's persistent personality forced us to keep working at a parenting style until we found what worked.

Hayden taught us that tiny babies don't manipulate, they communicate. A child psychologist friend who was visiting us was interested in Hayden's cry. She was impressed that the cry was not an angry, demanding one but rather an expectant one, as if Hayden knew she would be heard.

Hayden caused us to re-evaluate our job description as parents. We had always thought an effective parent needed to be in constant control. Then we realized that mind-set was self-defeating. It assumes that there is an adversarial relationship between parent and child: the baby is "out to get you", so you better get her first. Hayden made us realize our role was not to control her. It was to manage her, and to help her learn to control herself.

What helped us get over the fear-of-spoiling and the fear-of-being-manipulated mind-set was the realization that it was better to err on the side of being over-reactive and over-responsive. As we worked on developing a balance of appropriate responses, there were times when we responded too slowly and times when we jumped too quickly, but we felt that when in doubt, it was better to be responsive. Children who are perhaps indulged a bit (as many firstborn high-need children are) will at least develop a healthy self-image and trust in their parents. With this foundation it is easier to back off a bit as you try to create a healthy balance between parents' needs and child's. The child of parents who respond too little develops a poor self-image, and a distance develops between parent and child. This situation is harder to remedy. I have never heard parents in my paediatric practice say that they wish they hadn't held their baby so much. In fact, most, if able to rewind their parenting tape, would hold their baby more.

lesson

When in doubt, we listened and responded to her cries. She was trying to tell us something.

We also considered one of the earliest teachings that Martha had learned as a nurse and I had learned as a physician: first, do no harm (*primum non nocere*). We decided that if we tried to squelch Hayden's personality, we would be doing her harm and crippling her development. Our job as parents was not to change Hayden into a behavioural clone of every other baby. It would have been wrong to try to change her. (How dull the world would be if all babies acted the same!) It was better to widen our expectations and accept her the way she was, not the way we wished she was. Our parental role was like that of a gardener: we couldn't change the colour of the flower or the day when it would bloom, but we could pull the weeds and prune the plant so it blossomed more beautifully. Our role was to channel Hayden's behaviour and nurture her special qualities so that instead of being a liability, these temperament traits would later work to her advantage and serve her well.

lesson

Our job was to accept Hayden's unique personality, appreciate her special traits, and channel them into behaviour that would work for her, and for the family. It was not to change her for our own convenience.

Sleep, or rather the lack of it, became a major problem. Actually, for the first six months Hayden slept quite well, waking once or twice at night to be fed. She slept in a cradle right next to our bed, and when she stirred, Martha would nudge the cradle into motion or pat her. Unless she was hungry, she'd settle right back to sleep. Then Hayden learned to sit up, and the cradle was no longer safe. We replaced it with a cot up against the wall about twelve feet from our bed. Somehow she knew that was too far away, or maybe it was that the cot couldn't be nudged to rock. She woke more and more, until one night she was awake every hour. Martha said, "I don't care what the books say, I've got to get some sleep." Whereupon she nestled Hayden next to her in our bed. Once we discarded the picture of a self-soothing baby sleeping solo in a cot, we slept together happily.

lesson

Hayden was not a standard baby, and standard baby advice wouldn't work. Once we regarded her not as a behaviour problem to be fixed but as a personality to be nurtured, living with her became easier.

We found we had to be selective in choosing people with whom to commiserate. When we discussed our parenting dilemmas with friends, we came away feeling as if Hayden were the only baby in the whole wide world who couldn't satisfy herself during the day or settle herself at night. We concluded that no one could understand a baby like Hayden unless they'd had a baby like Hayden. Eventually, Martha found some like-minded mothers and surrounded herself with supportive friends. One of these women was a La Leche League leader who had recently moved to our community. A La Leche League group was started, and the mothers who came to the meetings gave and received valuable support.

lesson

We stopped complaining to people who didn't have a child like Hayden. Instead, we looked for support from people who truly understood our child and our parenting style.

what to call her

Hayden didn't fit any of the usual labels. She really wasn't a "fussy" baby, as long as we held her and attended to her needs. "Demanding", was just another way of saying, "spoiled". She wasn't "colicky", since she didn't seem to be in pain. Nor did the tag "difficult" ring true; some may beg to differ, but we were finding that holding and being near a baby to whom we were becoming so attached was not all that difficult. Besides, these labels were too negative for this little person who seemed to know so positively what she needed and how to get it. It wasn't until five years later, after talking with other parents of babies who also *needed* to feed so often, *needed* to be held a lot, *needed* human contact at night, that the term "high-need child" came to us. It best describes the kind of baby Hayden was and the level of parenting she needed.

In my paediatric practice, I discovered that the term "high-need child" was P.C. – psychologically correct. By the time drained parents came to me for counselling about their demanding baby, they had already been on the receiving end of a barrage of negatives: "You hold her too much." "It must be your milk." "She's controlling you." All this advice left parents with the underlying message of "bad baby because of bad parenting". They felt it was somehow their fault their baby acted this way. As soon as I offered the description "high-need child", I could see a look of relief on the faces of the parents. Finally, someone had something nice to say about their baby. "High-need" sounds special, intelligent, unique, and it shifts the focus to the baby's personality, relieving parents from the guilt of believing that their baby acts this way because of their parenting. Further, "high-need" suggests that there is something parents can do to help this baby. It underscores the idea that these babies simply need more: more touch, more understanding, more sensitivity, more creative parenting.

lesson

Redefining our baby in more positive terms helped us focus on her exciting qualities rather than her inconvenient ones.

our high-need child grew and changed

Needs change, but with Hayden her need level remained high. Hayden became a high-need toddler, then a high-need child, and we now tease her about being a "high-cost" teen. Her needs did not decrease as she grew; they merely changed (and so did our responses!)

Since as a baby Hayden did not willingly accept substitute care, we started something new in our town – we took our baby with us. With three older children, we had a lot of school meetings and events to attend, plus social gatherings with friends and hospital colleagues, sailing outings, church services, and so on. Everyone got used to seeing the three of us there.

Because she was breast-feeding, Martha could easily keep Hayden quiet when it was necessary. Usually, because her needs were satisfied, she was a joy to have around. No one objected to her presence. If it was obviously a "no kids" thing, we just didn't go.

We thought things would change when Hayden became a toddler, but we were definitely still in attachment-parenting training. We discovered that Hayden could sometimes be left with our thirteen-year-old, Jim, for short times,

because she was attached to him. But it didn't always work. We'd sometimes get called home when Jim's magic wore off too quickly. Hayden knew her level of tolerance for separation, and we learned not to exceed it.

One of our more vivid memories is that of frantic two-year-old Hayden running after us as we drove away. We stopped, even though we could see that Jim was right behind her, and reassessed our plans to go out alone. As we comforted her, listening carefully to her words and her expressions, we saw that her need to stay with us this time was much greater than our need to leave her behind. It was not hard for us to switch gears. Because of the way Hayden was able to communicate, we did not feel manipulated. The three of us set out together, feeling good about the way that we listened and were heard.

Yes, we occasionally felt a touch of doubt. "Are we creating an eternally dependent child who will never wean from us?" It's easy to feel that way, because you can see only a short distance into the future. Yet deep down we knew that what we were doing was right. We understood why at age two she couldn't stay in the nursery at church without one of us with her. When she still wouldn't at age three, we were embarrassed. Then, lo and behold, at three and a half she happily waved good-bye and didn't look back as she hurried off to her Sunday school class. What a relief to see her find her wings and experience church as a secure place to be because we had not forced her to be independent before she was ready. Hayden weaned from the breast at four years and from our bed at four and a half, when baby sister Erin

attachment parenting

Throughout this book you will read the term "attachment parenting". This is the parenting style that we began to learn with our first high-need baby and one that has proven to be a valuable management tool for high-need babies whose parents we have counselled. Attachment parenting is a high-touch, highly responsive way of caring for your baby that helps you feel close to your baby and your baby feel close to you. Consequently, your baby is able to cue his needs better and you are more intuitively able to read his cues and needs. It helps you and your baby get connected and helps you enjoy one another more. Actually, attachment parenting is not just for high-need babies. All babies need a higher level of attachment than our culture generally recognizes.

This style of parenting gets you and your baby off to the right start. By breast-feeding, carrying your baby a lot in a sling, and giving a nurturant response to your baby's cries, you gradually feel more comfortable and competent at baby care and more open to refining your style of parenting until you find what works best for you and your baby, without the fear of spoiling or being manipulated.

Attachment parenting is not an indulgent, unstructured, permissive style of childcare. On the contrary, it teaches parents how to respond *appropriately* to their child's needs, which includes knowing when to say no to the child and helping the child learn to manage her own needs. Attachment parenting begins with giving the infant roots, then helps her develop the wings to become independent, and ultimately gives her the tools to become a solid and secure person.

arrived. (Of course, we shared these milestones with only a few, select friends. Most assumed Hayden had crossed those bridges long ago.)

lesson

Hayden not only had higher needs, but they lasted longer.

her discipline needs were higher

We had been used to three compliant kids. When we held their hands, they turned in the direction we wished. With Hayden, we knew compliance would not come easily. Our earliest clue was her body language. Whenever we tried to redirect her impulse, her whole body would stiffen in resistance. We tried to turn her toward a safer activity; she turned toward the street. She was trying on her power. Back to the drawing board for discipline. As Hayden grew, it remained clear that we couldn't force our control over her – and should not try to. We needed to consider Hayden's sensitivity in disciplining her. This became more obvious as she got older, and she indicated to us that she needed to be given an active part in her own discipline. Any time we operated solely from our point of view, discipline was a dismal failure.

Hayden as a toddler was a determined explorer, and many times we would have to match her persistence with our own calm determination to stay in charge. When she reached for the knobs on the stereo, for example, we would matter-of-factly remove her to another place in the room and distract her with another activity. We had to repeat this redirection at least fifty times before she got the point. But even when she was only one year old, we felt it was important for us to command her respect.

Hayden's impulsiveness, we feared, would get her into trouble. She climbed up on furniture or counters only to realize she couldn't get down. Our knee-jerk reaction, rushing in to interrupt her climbing, only fed her determination, and hovering over her anxiously in these predicaments was enough to make her worry and be less surefooted. So, instead of letting our faces reflect our anxiety, we showed confidence in her ability to climb. Hayden picked up on our confidence in her; she realized that we, too, felt that she could handle the situation. We structured the environment so it was safe to climb, and then assumed the role of spotters,

being on standby to catch her if needed. The rest was up to her.

Sometimes it seemed wiser to under-react when Hayden was frustrated. As the first daughter, she was often being aggravated by her three older brothers. Yet we couldn't be rescuing her each time, nor would we have wanted to, since a certain amount of frustration is necessary for healthy development. So she developed "spunk" very early. If Hayden came running to her in distress, Martha would calmly say to her, "Do you need my help?" Usually Hayden managed on her own, knowing Martha would intervene if the aggravation developed into teasing or harassment.

The older Hayden got and the more experienced we became, the more confident we were in saying no to her. We believed that because she was a solid and secure child she could handle being thwarted at times and not having her needs instantly gratified. After all, the persistent personality of a high-need child sets her up for frustration, so she'd better learn how to handle setbacks.

lesson

Our job was not to prevent frustrations in Hayden's life, but rather to help her learn how to manage them.

Continuing to command Hayden's respect was one of our most difficult challenges at every stage of her development, and especially important when it came to the issue of talking back. When she became disrespectful toward

Martha, I would quickly intervene, "Hayden, I will not tolerate you talking like that, especially to someone I love."

It's easy for a child with a dominating personality to overpower the parents. Out of sheer exhaustion you give up, give in, and take the path of least resistance. Early on, we feared that because of her persistent personality Hayden would have difficulty accepting authority figures. (Our fears were later confirmed.) Dealing with Hayden was a constant contest of wits and wills. Sometimes we simply had to put on our parent-in-charge hat and say, "I'm the parent, you're the child, that's that!" Other times we had to walk with her for a while on her path before gradually rerouting her onto ours. This forced us to divide our conflicts into "biggies" (non-negotiable situations that required her compliance) and "smallies" (trivial, yet annoying, situations that threatened neither Hayden's respect for us nor her emerging self-image).

Early on we realized that learning to live with Hayden meant channelling her unique personality traits to work not only to her advantage but also to our advantage. Her keen awareness made her more sensitive to our moods, so we learned that when Hayden was being childish we had to be "adultish". Hayden taught us the concept of mirroring: children, especially hypersensitive ones, easily pick up their parents' moods. If a tantrum was about to erupt and we reflected an "it's okay, no problem" attitude, she would often mirror our peace and settle down. If we let ourselves get angry or worried about the tantrum, our anxiety just added fuel to her fire. When Hayden protested

our instructions and flew into a rage, we needed to stay calm. When she lost her self-control, we had to hang on to ours. If we lost our composure – and many times we did – it took twice as long for her to settle down. Acting like the adult in charge set a calmer mood that helped put a crumbling child back together.

lesson

As difficult as it was to do when Hayden became irritable to irritating, we had to maintain a peaceful presence.

We learned that with Hayden there were certain places that were not suitable for confrontations. (The problem with this insight was that we were often not disciplined enough ourselves to wait for a better time and place.) One of these times, as every parent knows, was mealtime. One of these places was the car. If Hayden felt pushed into a corner, she would typically lash out physically and hit or kick something. One memorable occasion was when she was in the front passenger seat. She was reacting strongly to something I was telling her. Knowing she tended to get physical, I should have backed off until we were in a less confined space, but I didn't. We still have the broken door on the glove compartment to remind us of that mistake.

Because Hayden was a challenge to our discipline skills, we were forced to get to know her in a way we had not experienced with our sons. The endless hours spent parenting Hayden produced a deep knowledge of who she was as a person, and this in turn helped her understand herself as a person. Rather than muzzling her, by responding to Hayden we rewarded her for being an expressive person. She became a master at expressing her needs and engaging the resources of adult caregivers at a very early age. She was a very resourceful three-year-old. The ability to express herself is an asset that will serve Hayden well as an adult.

As we watched Hayden dominate her peers in playgroups, we saw why she had earned the label "bossy". Like a quarterback addressing a huddle, she commanded all the kids' attention, and they lined up to listen as she told them how they were going to play the game. Now, we watch her dominate student council meetings in our living room, and we marvel at how she works on the members until they agree with her point of view.

Hayden early on caused us to re-evaluate the issue of control. We gradually figured out that the child shouldn't control the parents, or the parents control the child. Yet parents must control situations; when there is no limit-setting, family life is a disaster. We needed to be in charge of Hayden, to give her "house rules" and then control her environment so that it was not difficult for her to comply with these rules.

We were unprepared for the strong-mindedness we encountered in Hayden as a toddler. The older children had responded well to verbal cues. Hayden seemed not to hear us. So, rather than be constantly yelling "no, don't touch" (which was futile), we taught her that throughout the house there were "yes-touches" and "no-touches". Our job included making the "yes-touches" more accessible to her than the forbidden things. Hayden could operate from

her own inner controls in a setting that communicated order and structure of some sort. (Every family will do this differently.) When she had the opportunity to behave properly, independent of endless no's from us, she would start to get a sense of her own inner controls. When she's older and on her own, this set of inner rules will help her operate responsibly and confidently on her own. She'll feel right when she follows the rules and won't feel right when she doesn't. And we learned that in order to set limits and model desirable behaviour, we ourselves had to be disciplined.

lesson

Everything we did with and for Hayden from day one was discipline. We were teaching her the tools to succeed in life.

our needs versus her needs

Toward the middle of Hayden's first year, we realized that parenting a high-need child could have a better or worse effect on our relationship as husband and wife. Such a child can easily dominate the home. There were times when Martha risked burning out from over-giving. A warning sign of impending burnout was Martha saying: "I don't even have time to take a shower, Hayden needs me so much." For Martha's sake, and ultimately for the sanity of the whole family, I had to remind her, "What Hayden needs most is a happy, rested mother." It wasn't enough just to preach. Besides pitching in more around the house and with the older children, I took over with Hayden whenever I could. I would take her for a walk or car ride so that she would be out of Martha's sight and earshot.

lesson

As a mother, I realized I had to take good care of myself so I could take better care of my baby.

Having a high-need child helped us communicate more maturely with each other. There was always the "our needs versus her needs" dilemma. We had to steal time for ourselves, realizing that even the best parenting can be undermined if the marriage falls apart. I saw how important it was to Martha for me to validate her mothering. I frequently offered not only a reassuring "you know best", but when I saw that her drive to give was outpacing her energy reserves, I realized I needed to intervene and help. I sometimes wondered when I would ever have my wife back, but then realized we couldn't rewind this parenting tape. I was an adult, and Hayden would go through this stage only once.

From Martha's perspective, this balancing act was more easily said than done. There were plenty of times when I managed to let my own neediness send Martha double messages ("I've got needs, too, you know"). She would feel this pressure even when I thought I was doing a good job putting Martha's and Hayden's needs ahead of my own. And we both quickly found out that it

is difficult for some women to accept help with the responsibility of baby care even when they need it a lot. They often can't see that they need nurturing for themselves. Nor do they know how to make their own needs a high priority. We discovered that Martha was very good at taking care of everyone else but really did not know how to take care of herself. (We are still working on this seventeen years later.)

how we grew – the payoff

As Hayden grew, her neediness remained but her personality blossomed. One of the earliest qualities we noticed was her sensitivity, her ability to care and comfort when playmates were hurt or upset. As a preschooler, she had already developed a keen sense of justice and social values. Often she would say, "That's not right" or "How sad." Her love of people and her ability to connect with them was another payoff we witnessed. She would be aware of other children who needed mothering, and she would do what she could to help. Her sense of intimacy was appropriate, giving eye contact or a touch on the arm during a conversation. She had a confident way of being in the presence of adults. A child psychiatrist who was at our home one evening remarked, "Hayden knows where her body is in space." We knew what that meant. Because she had been held and nursed and responded to appropriately, Hayden already had a good sense of herself as a unique physical presence and she responded to others in their uniqueness. She was able even then to affirm each person she met. Since Hayden was used to being understood and responded to, she could express herself comfortably. This ability, combined with her high energy, caused us to joke about our "Sarah Bernhardt". It's no wonder that through her grade school and high school years, she enjoyed and excelled at being onstage. Her chosen course of study in college, if you haven't already guessed, is psychology and drama.

As Hayden matured as a person, we were maturing as parents. Gradually and subtly our parenting style, besides being nurturing to Hayden, became a source of growth for us. Hayden's high needs caused us to stretch ourselves to higher levels of giving with the ever-present challenge of balancing Hayden's needs with the rest of the family's. Hayden opened us up to be more flexible, more patient, and more disciplined. We came to realize that, although there are a few basic principles of good parenting that apply to every child and every temperament, how parents apply these principles is affected, for better or for worse, by the need level of the child. Compliant babies who can be put down in a cot while awake and who fall asleep on their own will accept a less intensive style of nighttime parenting. Compliant children will often switch gears from their agenda to their parents' at the slightest suggestion and come immediately when called to dinner from a distance. High-need children, on the other hand, need an eye-to-eye summons before switching from their agenda to yours.

Parenting high-need children has matured us as individuals, too. High-need children push buttons that reveal pleasant and unpleasant scenes from our childhoods. Parenting Hayden led us to make personal discoveries about how we ourselves were parented, and how this was affecting us as adults. When these flashbacks surfaced, we soon learned which ones we could use to our parenting advantage and which ones to discard, for example, the impulse to smack. Some people would have considered Hayden's behaviour cause for smacking, but we realized that she needed a different kind of "hands-on" discipline.

Hayden also caused our marriage to mature. We became very different partners as a result of our experience with parenting a high-need child. We knew that the best parenting requires two parents in the home. As tempting as it was for Martha to throw herself totally into mothering, she wisely directed some energy toward me. We have become much more sensitive to each other's temperaments and better at anticipating each other's needs. We have continued to avail ourselves of marriage-enrichment opportunities and plain old "enjoying time" together often.

Now that Hayden is about to leave the nest and enter college, we look back at our parenting with few regrets. We cannot take all the credit or blame for the person she becomes, yet it's comforting to know we gave her a good start. The rest is up to Hayden.

Hayden has gone from being a high-need child to a high-energy teen. Her life as a baby is chronicled in our earlier book *The Fussy Baby*. She sometimes opens that book and shows her friends, "That's me." One prom night, as she stood posed for her picture, she looked so grown up in her formal gown. I whispered to Martha, "Fussy baby fills out", and this mature teen-woman gave her daddy a wink. As she was escorted out the door, our minds and hearts filled with flashbacks of those countless energy-draining scenes of babyhood, toddlerhood, and childhood. Martha and I looked at each other and thought, "It's been a long and bumpy road, yet all that time in arms, at breast, and in our bed, the many discipline confrontations, and the years of high-touch parenting have produced a confident, compassionate, caring person. It has all been worthwhile."

chapter 2

profile of a high-need baby

"Why is my baby so different? She is not like any of my friends' babies. They sleep through the night. They're happy being held by anyone. My friends don't seem as tired as I am. What am I doing wrong?" Sound familiar? Your baby acts the way she does because that's the way she is. It's her personality.

In the first weeks after birth you get a glimpse of who this little person really is. Even while pregnant you may have had a hint of the challenge to come. High-need infants tend to be full-time tummy-thumpers and bladder-kickers, as if telling the world even before they're born that they need more space.

In some ways all babies are high-need babies, and most babies have high needs in at least one area of their life. Some have more high-need areas than others. All babies need attachment – high-need babies don't give up expressing this need. The neediness of the baby is often in the mind of the parent. Some experienced parents of children have widened their expectations of what babies are "normally" like, and they adapt more easily to a baby with high needs; new parents often are not so realistic. After Hayden introduced us to high-need babies, we learned a whole new way to parent. The babies that followed her each had their own particular high needs. We were able to recognize and respond to them because of our experience with Hayden. None of them were as thoroughly "high need" as Hayden, but they came close. In retrospect, we realize that the babies who came before Hayden had high needs, too, in some areas. The difference between those babies and Hayden was not only a difference in need levels; Hayden also had the forceful personality to let us know just what she needed. (Factored into our whole spectrum of parenting is that we were young and full of energy with the first babies. Hayden was born eleven years after our first child, Jim. By then we had less energy, perhaps, but more experience.)

We have met many high-need babies over the years. Based on this "gallery" we have compiled the following profile of a high-need baby. All babies will show some of these features some of the time, and these features are descriptive only. As you will see, each of these personality traits has its blessings and its trials. These personality traits should not be judged as good or bad. They simply show differences among babies; but these differences do make high-need babies challenging to parent. Ultimately, what matters is how the child learns to use these special gifts. Our goal is to help parents identify these unique features in their infant and channel these traits to work to their child's advantage.

intense

"He's going to be a handful", one midwife said to another as they tried to console newborn baby George. You can often spot high-need babies in the hospital. Even at a few hours of age, George had an instinct about what he needed *and* the persistence required to get it. The cry of a high-need baby is not a mere request; it's an urgent demand. These babies put more energy into everything they do. They cry loudly, feed voraciously, laugh with gusto, and protest more forcefully if their needs are not met. Because they feel everything so deeply, they react more powerfully if their feelings are disturbed. "If I don't feed him as soon as he fusses, he falls apart" is a common statement from the mother of such a baby.

You can read the intensity of the baby's feelings in her body language. The fists are clenched, back arched, muscles tensed, as if ready for action.

I set up a cradle in our room so we could hear Mara's cries at night. It quickly became clear that not only would we be able to hear her, so would everyone on the block. Mara was LOUD! When she started crying, it would quickly escalate. The intensity and shrillness sounded as if something must be very wrong. We would feed her, burp her, change her, rock her, walk with her, but sometimes nothing seemed to help. After a while, I found myself going into overdrive instantly whenever she cried, because I knew if it got out of control she'd quickly disintegrate, and it would take her a long time to come back around. I became obsessive in trying to prevent her from getting upset in any way because there was hell to pay if she did. She was a type A personality right from birth.

Intense babies become intense toddlers, characterized by one word: "driven". They seem in high gear all the time. Their drive to explore and experiment with everything within reach leaves no household item safe. Some high-need toddlers manoeuvre around the house carefully, but most do not. Most of these babies run headlong toward a desired object, seemingly oblivious of everything in their path. Soon it dawns on you that the same behavioural trait that can exhaust you will also delight you. The same drive that gets your toddler into trouble also leads him to a level of creativity that other children may not venture to reach. Your job is to help him drive carefully on roads that he can handle.

can you make a child high-need?

We believe that most high-need children are born with this trait. In fact, all babies have high needs for being held and comforted, but some babies are able to express their needs more strongly than others because they haven't shut down (withdrawn) due to the trauma of separation. Some critics believe that parents make their child needy by how they parent. The great majority of parents we have counselled brought their high-need babies into the world and followed their own intuitive parenting to give their child the level of care he needed. This is healthy behaviour which will work to the advantage of parent and child. On occasion, however, we see a "helicopter mother", who hovers over the child and anxiously responds within a millisecond to the child's every whim. This is unhealthy for both mother and child. The mother's needs for intimacy are being met by her doting over her child, and the child uses the perceived neediness to control the mother. In extreme cases, the child is crippled by not learning self-management skills. This parent needs professional counselling.

hyperactive

This feature of high-need babies, and its cousin, hypertonic, are directly related to the quality of intensity. The term "hypertonic" refers to muscles that are frequently tensed and ready to go, tight and waiting to explode into action. The muscles and mind of high-need children are seldom relaxed or still. "Even when he was a newborn, I could feel the wiry in him", one mother related. "She hated being swaddled", another mother volunteered. Most infants, even high-need ones, welcome being wrapped in a blanket, worn in a sling, or draped over your shoulder to mould into the contour of your body, but there are some high-need babies who seem to shun containment and physical restraint. They stiffen their limbs and arch their backs when you try to hold them, and they are frequently seen doing back dives in your lap, turning even breast-feeding into a gymnastic event.

Parents, remember that, like all the words used to describe high-need children, the term "hyperactive" is not a negative tag. At what point a normally active child becomes a hyperactive child is a judgment call. Calling your busy toddler hyperactive does not mean he will be burdened with this label forever, or that a school psychologist will someday tag him "hyperactive". This term just describes how your child acts, without making any judgment about whether it's good or bad. Hyperactive in an infant or toddler is not a disorder, it's a description.

"Hyper" is often in the eye of the child-watcher. Activity level is relative to the company the child keeps. Place an intense, creative, enthusiastic child in the midst of a group of more reserved children, and the doer gets tagged "hyper". Also, the activity level of the child depends on the setting. A child may play quietly in the comfortable, known environment of his own home, yet be frantic and undirected in a playgroup full of strangers.

"There's no such thing as a still shot", said one photographer-father of a high-need baby. "His motor seems stuck in fast idle", another father commented. These motor traits are part of the baby's personality. They may be hard to live with at times, but this restlessness is not necessarily a negative trait. Many highly creative, world-changing people were labelled hyperactive as children.

draining

High-need babies extract every bit of energy from tired parents – and then want more. Though parents use the term "draining", it's not an apt description. What you give your baby doesn't go down the drain. Perhaps "siphoning" is a more accurate term, because what you are really doing is transferring much of your energy into your baby's tank to help her thrive. You will need to muster up as positive an attitude as you can; try to think of these draining days as giving days. This will help get you through those high-maintenance early months.

Babies take the fuel they need from you without considering whether they leave anything behind in mother's gas tank. The seemingly constant holding, feeding, and comforting leave little energy for your needs. Experienced mothers learn to operate in what one woman calls "the mother zone" (like the *Twilight Zone*); you feel a bit fuzzy, somewhat sleep-deprived; you simply function in low gear for a stretch of time. It's a season that passes; and while you're in it, try not to fight it or resent it.

communication, not control

One of the most difficult mental adjustments for parents to make is overcoming the fear of "being manipulated" and "losing control". Once you make the switch in mind-set to believing that your baby is communicating her needs, not controlling your lives, thriving and surviving with a high-need baby will be much easier.

Instead of feeling sorry for yourself that you didn't get enough sleep, just don't expect as much from yourself that day. Of course you're not completely rested – you are the mother of a baby who needs you. Time spent in the mother zone is good for you and for baby. Ease up on yourself and you'll be easier to be around. You'll be happier getting less done. Other tasks can wait, but baby can't.

Many mothers seem to have an internal energy gauge that magically brings in more fuel just as the tank nears empty. There will be days of incessant holding with no breaks. But just when you feel you can't cope with another day of giving, you get a second wind, and suddenly you can relax and enjoy your baby's unique personality blooming. Perhaps baby even senses mother's breaking point and backs off a bit. There probably won't be any days off, but some days will be less difficult than others.

feeds frequently

You will soon learn that feeding is not only a source of nutrition, but also an easy tool for comforting, not only because the skin-to-skin contact makes the breast a nice place to nestle, but also because the baby can easily regulate the flow of milk. Studies show that babies who are fed frequently, as needed, cry less than infants who are fed on a more rigid, parent-controlled schedule. In cultures in which babies rarely cry, as documented, for example, in Liedloff's *The Continuum Concept*, infants usually breast-feed twenty or so times a day. Researchers have attributed the mellowness of the babies in these "higher" cultures to the effect frequent feeding has on the overall organizing of the baby's biological systems. This number of feedings sounds incredible to us in our Western culture, but it's really not so strange when you consider that in these cultures baby is worn on the mother's body in such a way that he has easy access to the breast. A feeding in this case may

the "velcro" mother and baby

Tracy and her baby, Michael, seemed to be constantly attached. In fact, when Michael was one month of age, Tracy tagged him "the Velcro baby". You never saw one without the other. When Michael wasn't nursing at Tracy's breasts, he was in her arms or in her sling. When Tracy worked about the house, she wore Michael in her sling, a scene she called "work and wear". On particularly high-need days, Tracy said, "I seem to put him on in the morning and take him off at night." When Michael wasn't on some part of Tracy's body, he was glued to Daddy. This baby was put down only for a long nap, when Tracy needed to attend to her personal needs, or when he grew up enough to demand some "floor time". At night, baby and mother did not go their separate ways either. The pair slept face-to-face, tummy to tummy, nursing several times at night without either member of the pair fully awakening. Not all babies need this much intensive care, and not all mothers are comfortable providing it, but for many high-need families, this level of attachment works smoothly, especially when they realize that this high-maintenance stage does not last forever.

As a parent, you'll put your hours in at one end or the other of the time your child lives with you. We personally would much rather put that time in when they are infants and toddlers than when they are teens. Our teens have not given us the chance to find out what it would be like to sit up all night wondering where they are or whom they're with. But we can imagine this would be far more nerve-racking than being there for our infants and toddlers when they need us so much.

last only five minutes, rather than the thirty to forty-five minutes a baby takes to fill his tummy when fed only six or eight times a day in a more controlled feeding arrangement.

We live in a culture that is definitely at odds with this "primitive" style of mothering. And our babies cry a lot! It is a challenge to a Western mother of a high-need baby to find a lifestyle that both she and her baby can live with. And there must be a balance in feeding. Overfed formula-feeders can get fat, so using a formula-filled bottle as a constant pacifier is certainly not healthy or appropriate. The good news is, you don't have to worry about over-breast-feeding, because the caloric content of breast milk self-adjusts to frequent feeding; when baby has just a brief "comfort-feed", she gets only the lower-calorie foremilk. Besides, frequent breast-feeders rarely remain overweight, even if for a while some look like miniature sumo wrestlers. Studies show that the fat cells laid down by breast-feeding babies are quite different from those of babies fed manufactured baby milk. The fat melts away once baby becomes mobile. So how often should you breast-feed your high-need baby? As frequently as baby needs, yet not to the extent that it wears you out. There are other ways to comfort high-need babies, and it's important to learn some of these alternatives.

We're in harmony with each other. I nurse an average of eighteen times a day. I know this sounds like a lot of nursing, but there is never a schedule to it. Either she lets me know or I just start it. It always works out. Nursing is never a hassle or bother. It's just second nature to me. I don't even think about it or worry about it. It

first-class baby

A lot of this book was written in the peace and quiet of coast-to-coast flights during a year of frequent public speaking. On one flight, when I was fortunate to be upgraded to first class, I identified with a high-need baby who "has it made". He gets a higher standard of care – he goes first class! The high-need baby gets held more because he protests if he is put down. The high-need baby gets fed more because he demands it. He (usually) enjoys the first-class comfort of sleeping with his parents because he refuses to sleep separate. And, he gets taken to more interesting places because he is unwilling to accept a lower level of care. For high-need babies, life is one continuous upgrade.

seems like we are always in harmony. We just nurse whenever or wherever Lindsey or I start it.

"Schedule" is not in the high-need baby's vocabulary. Early on, these smart infants learn that the breast or bottle is not only a source of nutrition, but also a source of comfort. In fact, research has shown that non-nutritive sucking (sucking for comfort rather than for food) is one of the earliest ways a baby learns to settle. Mothers figure this out quickly and, unfortunately, many of them get their babies hooked on dummies so they can be put down, away from mother, a lot. We prefer that mother use her own finger to give baby extra suck time if he is bottle-fed, or if she knows he doesn't need any more milk from her breast, or if her breasts need a break.

A recurrent theme that we hear from the parents of high-need babies is "She wants to feed all the time." Martha's experience with Hayden is a perfect example. Because our first three babies went an average of three hours between feedings – or even four hours once we added solid food to their diet in the early months – she expected the same from Hayden. Her approach with the first three was to feed them when they cried. But when Hayden cried one hour after being fed, she wondered what to do. Of course, feeding is what Hayden needed, Martha discovered. Yet how could this be? She spent two weeks charting Hayden's feeding habits in an effort to see what sort of schedule she had. At the end of the two weeks she looked at the chart and concluded that this baby simply didn't have a schedule. That's when Martha adopted the slogan "go with the flow".

Expect baby's need to nurse to intensify during high-need days when baby will naturally gravitate toward her favourite pacifier and person, which to a breast-fed baby is one and the same. Yes, you will feel like a human dummy or "pacifier", because you are. Yet, consider that "pacifier" means "peacemaker". Certainly this is the ultimate goal of parenting the high-need baby: to give this growing infant an internal peace during those tumultuous months after birth, when baby is learning to settle into life; this will help her learn to create inner peace on her own.

Nursing is a wonderful time-out when we are both wearing thin. It alleviates a tightened clash of the wills and provides a calm and loving oasis where we are both refreshed. I am always grateful for prolactin [the breast milk–producing hormone that has a relaxing effect on mother].

Not only do high-need babies breast-feed more frequently, the need for breast-feeding lasts longer. These babies are notoriously slow to wean. They realize that they have a good thing going and that it would be foolish to give it up quickly. It is not unusual for high-need babies (unless forced to wean before their time) to breast-feed at least two years. (See weaning, pages 150–1, for how extended feeding benefits mother and child.)

demanding

High-need babies don't merely request feeding and holding, they demand it – loudly. This personality trait more than any of the others pushes parents' buttons, causing them to feel manipulated and controlled. Adults who are stuck in the "parenting equals control" mind-set may have great difficulty realizing that baby's demands equal communication, not control.

Mothers of high-need babies often say, "I just can't get to him fast enough." These babies convey a sense of urgency in their signals; they do not like waiting, and they do not readily accept alternatives. Woe to the parent who offers baby the rattle when he is expecting a breast. He will let you know quickly and loudly that you've misread his cues. The concept of "delayed gratification" is totally foreign to infants. It must be sensitively and gradually taught when the child is developmentally ready to learn it.

It may be easier to cope with your baby's demanding signals if you understand why high-need babies have to be demanding in order to thrive. Suppose baby had high needs but did not have a strong personality to "demand" that these needs get met. Suppose he did not use the kind of persistent cry that ensures a response. This would be a lose-lose situation: baby would not thrive because his needs would not be met, and parents would not get enough practice at cue reading to ever pick up on the baby's real need level.

If the child feels that she can trust her caregivers, she will eventually learn to make her demands in a more socially acceptable way, rather than overwhelming the whole care-giving environment. With parents who both respond to and wisely channel her demands, the high-need child develops into a person with determination, one who will fight for her rights. The child becomes a leader instead of a follower, one who does not just follow the path of least resistance and do what everyone else is doing. Certainly, our country needs more such citizens.

Although being demanding is the trait of high-need children that is most likely to drive parents bananas, it is also the trait that drives children to succeed and excel. A high-need child with a demanding personality will, if nurtured and channelled appropriately during the formative years, exhaust teachers as she did her parents; yet she will also be able to extract from adult resources, such as teachers, the level of help and education she will need to thrive in academic and social endeavours. This is why it is so important not to squelch an infant's expressiveness. The ability to know one's needs and be able to express them comfortably is a valuable tool for success in life.

As the high-need infant grows into a high-need toddler and child, parents must also help her learn that her demands have to be balanced against the needs of others, so that she can learn to be a likable and compassionate person. Helping a demanding infant develop persistence without becoming a controlling person is one of the challenges we will discuss throughout this book.

awakens frequently

"Why do high-need babies need more of everything but sleep?" groaned a tired mother. You would think that high-need babies would need more sleep; certainly their tired parents do. In Chapter 8 we will explain why high-need children sleep differently, and offer nighttime parenting tips for you and your baby. To remedy your own tired feelings, remember what we said previously about living in the "mother zone".

I have gradually come to realize that she just doesn't need to sleep, and I can't force her to do so. The best thing I can do is to continue to provide a nurturing environment conducive to sleep and realize that she will eventually sleep more and so will I.

channelling behaviour versus changing behaviour

Channelling behaviour starts with knowing and accepting the child that you have been given. You use your knowledge of your child's behaviour to structure your home environment and shape your interactions with your child in such a way that the child's behavioural traits blossom to his advantage, as well as to his family's and society's. This is much healthier and more successful than trying to change your child's basic nature, trying to reshape him into a behavioural clone of everyone else. High-need children whose behaviour is channelled appropriately may be the leaders of the future. In fact, many people who have contributed positively to society were once high-need children whose behaviour was gently shaped by wise and sensitive parents. Many people who have grown up to harm society have been high-need children who were not recognized or nurtured. A high need that is unmet may reappear later as a less healthy need, one that is difficult to meet in a socially acceptable fashion. A high need that is met early is more likely to reappear later as a positive quality for the child, one that works to his advantage. A mother who recognized early that she had a high-need infant and worked hard to channel that child's behaviour confided to me, "Early on, I knew this child had the potential to be either a criminal or President."

unsatisfied

Not being able to satisfy a baby's needs is very frustrating for parents of high-need babies. It seems like a direct attack on your abilities. After all, isn't a contented baby the hallmark of effective mothering? Wrong! There will be days when you feed, rock, walk, drive, wear, and try every comforting technique known to man or woman, and nothing will work. Don't take this as a sign of failure. You do the best you can, and the rest is up to the baby. You have not failed as a mother even if your baby is miserable much of the time. This is partly his personality and partly his immature nervous system still in need of being organized. Meanwhile, keep experimenting with one comforting tool after another, and you will eventually discover one that works – at least for that day. Then you will feel like a genius! Keep your detective hat on to find clues to your baby's discomfort (see pages 138 and 162). Constant trial and error is how you build up your baby-soothing abilities.

unpredictable

It's frustrating to realize that what worked yesterday doesn't work today. "Just as I think I am winning, he ups the stakes", a baffled mother confided. High-need babies are inconsistently appeased because their nervous systems are poorly organized. You will need lots of variety in your bag of comforting tricks.

Rocking, walking, using carriers, singing lullabies, tummy position, back position, side position, infant seats, dummies, tilting the mattress of the bed, bringing him to bed with us, cuddling him on breasts or bare chest, bathing

your baby's temperament

"Temperament" describes the basic emotional wiring of your baby. How your baby expresses her unique wiring is through her personality. What kind of person your child becomes depends on her inborn temperament (nature) and your responses to it (nurture). Temperament is not "good" or "bad"; it is simply the way your baby is. A vital part of living with your baby's temperament is to know how to respond to it. There will be times you need to mellow a fussy baby or perk up a laid-back one.

It's important to know not only the temperament of your baby but yours too. Parent and baby need to find a way to fit. This little word so economically describes the relationship between parent and baby. Some pairs fit together more easily, while some mothers and fathers and their babies have to make a few adjustments along the way to improve the fit. If your baby has high needs and a persistent personality that demands that those needs be met, and you are a person who loves to be in control and to have your life run in a smooth, predictable routine, you and your baby will both have to do some

adjusting. It may be easier for a laid-back mother who by nature "goes with the flow" to cope with the unpredictable demands of a high-need baby.

The goal of parenting a high-need baby is to allow baby and parent to *shape each other's behaviour* so that personalities mesh rather than clash, and eventually you will bring out the best in each other.

A responsive, flexible, nurturing mother is a good match for a high-need baby. This baby challenges the mother's abilities and keeps her interested in her job, while the mother mellows the baby's temperament by helping her feel right most of the time. The attachment style of parenting really pays off in developing a good fit. The hours you spend each day in high-touch, responsive parenting will naturally help you and your baby fit. Initially, you may have to work at it, but you will be surprised how the fit develops naturally – as long as you practise a responsive style of parenting that lets it happen. When mother and infant fit, they will roll smoothly along the road of life together; if they fit poorly, the road is likely to be bumpy.

him just before sleep time, hot water bottles wrapped inside a fake fur animal, letting him stay awake until midnight before bedtime routines, starting right after dinner, letting him cry, not letting him cry – nothing seemed to work. Some of these things worked some of the time; nothing worked all the time. This is very frustrating; you wonder what you are doing wrong.

Along with their unpredictability, these children show extremes of mood swings. When happy, they are a joy to be around; they are master charmers and people pleasers. When angry, they let everyone around them feel the heat.

The child's unpredictability makes your day unpredictable. Do you take him shopping and risk a mega-tantrum when his first grocery grabs are thwarted, or will this be a day when he is the model shopping-trolley baby, charming everyone at the checkout counter?

When he is happy, he is the happiest baby around, but when he is angry he is the worst baby around. He is still that way, sunshine and smiles, anger and daggers. He has no middle emotion.

We have a theory that certain types of children show up in families that have certain areas in which they need to grow. When Hayden came along, our life had settled into a level of predictability that was quite comfortable, possibly heading for the "stale" category. We had three sons, easygoing types who liked sports and eagerly marched to the beat of the drummer in our family (Bill). We had similar interests professionally – we worked in paediatric

settings, pursued writing together, and Martha's interest in childbirth education and breast-feeding counselling fitted right into our paediatric setting. If Hayden hadn't come along to introduce us to unpredictability, our work as authors would probably have begun and ended with one book (and even that one book might have turned out to be "plain vanilla"). Meeting the challenge of this "different" baby forced us to discover our creative selves. Hayden taught us that life with a high-need child is never boring.

supersensitive

High-need babies are keenly aware of the goings-on in their environment. "Easily bothered", "quickly stimulated", "like walking on eggshells" is how parents describe their sensitive babies. High-need babies prefer a secure and known environment, and they are quick to protest when their equilibrium is upset. They startle easily during the day (for example, we learned not to turn on the blender if Hayden was anywhere nearby) and settle with difficulty at night. While you can carry on normal family life without waking most sleeping infants, these babies often awaken at the slightest noise. These supersensitive infants are unlikely to accept substitute caregivers willingly.

This acute sensitivity to their environment can become a rewarding asset as a high-need child grows. These children are more "tuned in" to what is going on around them. Their keen awareness stimulates their curiosity, which in turn stimulates learning. They are not distant

strive for balance

Many new mothers and fathers start parenting believing they must be in control of their child. Or, they may be the product of controlling parents themselves and have vowed not to do anything to squelch their child's personality. Both extremes cripple a child. Putting the lid on a child's personality stunts the child's emotional growth. Letting a child's emotions and character traits go unguided risks having the child turn out wild and lacking in self-control. Aim for a balance. Children need to be comfortable expressing their needs, yet high-need children need a high level of guidance to express themselves appropriately.

For the sake of your child, and yourself, in the early weeks of parenting, unload the baggage of your "control mind-set" and learn to give freely. When you have opened yourself up to be flexible enough to keep working at a style of parenting that helps all family members thrive, control will no longer be an issue. Without the stifling baggage of control hindering your intuitive parenting, you will be free to guide your child, channelling his personality traits to work to his advantage and to the advantage of the family.

children. They become kids who care, more easily bothered by another child's hurts. Most develop empathy, a quality that is lacking in many of today's teens and adults. Because these children are so sensitive, they develop great discernment and are able to consider the effects of their behaviour on the feelings of others. They are able to achieve one of the ultimate qualities of self-discipline: the ability to think through what they're about to do.

Supersensitive babies react in a big way to physical and emotional discomforts. They let you know, in no uncertain terms, they hurt and they need help – now!

He cries in protest when the littlest thing is not right with him. He is so sensitive. Whenever he has a cold, he cries and whines, and needs to be held constantly. He wails when he has an ear infection. At his nine-month check-up, I recall our paediatrician saying, "Wow! So much anger for such a little baby." I think he was just angry that his teeth hurt.

Though upsetting to your ears and frustrating to your sensitive heart, supersensitive babies are at least easier to read. They let you know when they need help or when something should be changed in their care-giving environment. Their signals cannot go unnoticed.

traits with a silver lining

A unique feature of high-need children is that what appears to be a "negative" personality trait can turn out to be positive. For every hour of sleep you lose in the early years, you are likely to get an extra hour of sleep when the child is a teen. For every ounce of distress the infant gives you, you are likely to get back at least an equal amount of delight. The same behavioural traits that earn these infants various negative labels are the ones that help their personality blossom. Early on, it's normal for parents to be overwhelmed with the negatives: loss of freedom, loss of sleep, and loss of energy. (See Chapter 7, "Mother Burnout".) Yet the sooner you can turn these negative attitudes into positive ones, the easier living with your high-need child will become. Don't think of your child as a difficult sleeper; think of her as active or alert. Don't think of him as clingy; think of him as a baby who values being with you. This is a tough challenge, one that requires self-discipline, but the rewards are great. Try to spend as much of your day focusing on the uniqueness of your child, identifying and reinforcing the child's positive character traits so that they will work to the child's advantage, and to yours. In addition, you'll get the added bonus of learning, by necessity, to take better care of yourself – a life skill that will benefit your whole family.

unable to be put down

High-need babies crave touch: skin-to-skin contact in your arms, at your breasts, in your bed. They extract whatever physical contact they can from their caregivers. They also crave motion. Holding is not enough; the holder must keep moving. If the holder wants to sit down, it had better be on something that rocks, glides, or swings. This constant holding may be particularly difficult for new parents who expected to have the magazine-model baby, the one who lies quietly in the cot gazing at fancy mobiles. This is not the play profile of the high-need baby. Parents' arms and bodies are his cot; mother's breasts are his pacifier; and a bouncing lap is his chair. Most high-need babies choose to upgrade their accommodations from the cot or playpen to the baby sling. They like to be worn many hours a day because they like the physical contact and they like to be up where the action is. Smart babies.

uncuddly

While most high-need babies are super-cuddly and crave being held, some are slower to warm up and often receive the label "uncuddly". It could be that this behaviour is caused by extreme sensitivity, which causes them to perceive handling as unsettling or threatening. It is important for the parent to stay calm and relaxed. Babies like this need careful handling that avoids over-stimulation and gradually desensitizes them to touch. Eventually, most will become accustomed to relaxed touching and holding. Some uncuddly babies continue to resist close physical contact, being closely contained in the sling, or spending long periods of time in one person's arms. They also protest being swaddled. These are the babies who need more space and floor time. The uncuddly babies are the most difficult of high-need babies because they don't melt and mould rewardingly into the arms of their caregivers. If you have a baby who is initially uncuddly, don't take it personally. These babies are simply slower to warm up to physical contact. Many of them eventually ease into the high-touch style of parenting that their high-need colleagues have learned to enjoy.

From the beginning Gennie seemed to be extremely sensitive. After nursing, she would pull away from me. At night she did not want to be touched at all. She would not make eye contact with anyone. When she began to smile or "talk", it was only to inanimate objects (like a doll) at first.

I felt her withdrawal from people was a problem. At night I began by putting one of my fingers against her arm while she slept. Over the weeks I progressed slowly, adding more touch until she no longer withdrew. I held her as much as possible during the day. I arranged my schedule so that I had to be out only two days and spent the rest of *the week at home. Some of those days I barely got dressed by noon. We rocked, read, and nursed.*

As Gennie learned to accept touch, she seemed to need it even more than the norm. I held her as much as possible. I learned quickly how much she needed me. Gennie liked her dad just fine – as long as mum was there! She really did not relate to outsiders until she was three or four years old.

the perfect match of needs and temperament

In order for children's high needs to work to their long-term advantage, their outward personality must accurately reflect their inner need level. Suppose an infant is born needing to be held a lot, fed frequently, and responded to in a consistent, nurturing manner. (Actually, all babies are like this.) Suppose that infant also has a rather laid-back personality and seems to be an "easy" baby. This baby would be at a disadvantage because his body language would convey that he did not need to be held much. On the other hand, a baby whose high need level is matched with a persistent, expressive personality will get what he needs. His cries will demand a response, and his compelling body language will ensure that he is picked up, held, and fed. Although more exhausting to parents, this baby is more likely to thrive because his need level is reflected in a personality that knows how to get those needs met.

not a self-soother

Another unrealistic expectation many new parents have is that babies will soothe themselves to sleep with the help of a dummy, a musical box, or some baby-calming gadget. High-need babies won't accept that. They need to interact with people, not things. Parents will often report, "He just can't relax by himself." Most babies need help to fall asleep. A parent who rocks, jiggles, walks, or dances with a baby at bedtime acts like a shock absorber for the day's stimulation and frustration. High-need babies must learn to trust their parents to help them. This will help them learn to relax on their own, a skill that has value for a lifetime. Crying oneself off to sleep is not a good way to learn to relax. The best way for a baby to learn to relax and fall asleep is to have his behaviour shaped for him by a parent. Once a child learns to relax on his own, he'll have no trouble falling asleep on his own.

The quality of wanting people instead of things as comforters, while initially exhausting, will eventually work to the child's advantage. The child will have a better grasp on interpersonal relationships, especially being comfortable with the quality of intimacy. (See the related section on intimacy on page 219.)

We learned early on that Amy was a people person. She preferred anything human to anything synthetic or mechanical. We tried a host of different things designed to soothe or entertain small infants, but Amy would have none of them. At our childbirth class reunion, all the other babies seemed quiet and content, sitting in infant seats or lying peacefully on the floor. Amy wanted and needed to be in our arms. That day, we got a lot of suggestions about ways to help her. Many other parents were extolling the virtues of the mechanical swing, telling of the many hours their baby would spend in it. Babies who had not tried one were put in the host's swing and almost always promptly fell asleep. We dutifully tried Amy in it and she cried immediately. Over the months that followed, we learned in no uncertain terms that she preferred arms to the cradle and the breast to the bottle. We came to respect this tendency in her. The pushchair, the cradle, the infant seats were all put away until she signalled that she was ready to be more physically separate from us. Now, at nearly a year old, she sleeps peacefully on a futon at naptime and loves taking rides in the pushchair and backpack. That time of needing intense physical contact was quite short. We're proud that we were able to be there for her in the way that she needed us to be.

separation-sensitive

The song "Only You" could be the theme of most high-need babies. These infants do not readily accept substitute care and are notoriously slow to warm up to strangers. As a mother of a clingy baby described it, "Amanda didn't like new people or new places and seemed to be in a continual phase of separation anxiety. Baby-sitters wouldn't watch her because of her reputation as a screamer. This was hard on me because I desperately needed a break from the intensity of my child."

better early than late

Needs that are met early in life go away. Needs that are left unmet never entirely disappear. Instead, the child can follow one of several paths. He can go through life with lower expectations and resign himself to an unfulfilled life. He can spend his life coping on his own and never learn to use the resources of others. Or, he can live a life of anger that the responses he expected were not the responses he got. He will always be searching without really knowing what he is searching for. It's a case of "parent me now" or "parent me later". Therapists' offices are filled with high-need adults in search of re-parenting.

It helps to see separation from the baby's viewpoint. To most adults, especially those of the "babies must learn to be independent" mind-set, baby and mother should be separate people, able to function on their own. Babies don't see it that way. In their minds, mother is a part of them, and they are part of mother. Mother and baby are one, a complete package. These babies feel right when they feel at one with mother; they feel anxious and frightened when not with mother. Adults dub this completely normal behaviour "separation anxiety". In reality, these emotions are normal feelings inside a little person who knows that he needs the presence of his mother to thrive and to feel complete. Labels such as "stranger anxiety" or "separation anxiety" are adult jargon, reflecting our expectations of how we want

babies to act for our own convenience, not how babies really are, or what they really need.

We have observed that mothers who spend the early months practising what we call attachment parenting (wearing their baby many hours a day in a sling, breast-feeding on cue, taking their babies with them wherever they go, and often sleeping with baby) themselves experience separation anxiety when not with their baby. If this anxiety appears in normal mothers, shouldn't it also be normal in babies? Fortunately, high-need babies have powerful personalities to tell us when things are not right.

Your baby's quality of being very selective about who cares for her shows that she is highly discerning. High-need babies know which situations and which people they can trust to meet their needs, and they protest if these expectations are not met. Loud separation protests also reveal that these babies have a capacity for forming deep attachments – if they didn't care deeply, they wouldn't fuss so loudly when separated. This capacity is the forerunner of intimacy in adult relationships.

Eventually, the infant's care-giving circle will grow to include people other than mother. The concept of weaning can be applied to more areas than just the breast or bottle. It also means letting go of exclusive relationships. When a new baby comes along, for example, the older one by necessity must begin to wean from mother to father (if she hasn't started already). Our own high-need babies were willing to stay happily with people other than Martha by age three and a half, and sooner than that if that person was someone to whom they were already strongly attached (father, sibling, close friend of mother's,

growing out of it

Will he ever stop fussing? Will she ever sleep through the night? When will the colic stop? Will I ever get my wife back? The good news is that, yes, babies do grow out of their difficult-to-manage behaviours and grow into more manageable ones. Write the following survival motto on a piece of paper and hang it on your wall: THIS TOO WILL PASS.

There are many milestones in the first two years of a child's life that bring with them improvements in behaviour and feelings of relief for parents. Within a month, babies can see images a foot away quite clearly, allowing baby to be soothed by eye-to-eye contact with a familiar, caring face. Increasing visual acuity between one to three months allows babies to be happily distracted by moving objects at increasing distances; watching a hand move or their reflection in a mirror will fascinate them. The first truly magical turning point is around three to four months, when many babies enter the promised land of fuss-free living. (High-need babies just don't get very far across the border!) At this age, they often develop more internal organization of their sleeping and waking patterns. The ability to see clearly across the room can be distracting enough that they forget to fuss. Also, between three and four months some babies find their thumb to soothe themselves, and all of them discover the entertainment value of their hands and fingers. Between four and six months, babies lie on their backs, kicking their legs in delight, enjoying their ability to make purposeful movements. This increasing neurological organization helps babies gain control over their bodies and use their hands and limbs for soothing and entertaining themselves.

Between six and nine months, babies begin to sit up by themselves and progress from sitting to crawling. This may be the first time that you are able to set your baby down and enjoy a few minutes of having both arms free. As babies' motor skills start to take off, they begin to literally move out of their upsetting behaviour. From nine to twelve months, the ability to pick up objects using the thumb and forefinger together broadens babies' play and feeding skills. They can do many more things all by themselves.

The next major turning point comes between twelve and eighteen months, when babies begin to walk, and then to run and climb. Babies' increasing ability to get around on their own means they drain less energy from you because they can do more to entertain and help themselves. This is a good time, weather permitting, to spend as much time outdoors as you can. Park yourself on a blanket under a tree with a good book and let baby explore in a safely enclosed area. In bad weather, spread the blanket indoors. You might manage to do some reading, and the two of you will have a better time when you don't spend all day trying to "get something done". Now is the time when you can get things done if you figure out a way to have baby be a part of the action. Whether you are cleaning house, gardening, or paying bills, toddlers are ecstatic if they can imitate you.

One of the highest energy-output stages in child rearing comes between fourteen and eighteen months. This is the time to draft some well-nurtured four- to six-year-olds to play with your toddler. They have tremendous energy for entertaining a baby, and you get to relax and simply supervise.

From eighteen to twenty-four months, language skills emerge, allowing the toddler to begin expressing frustrations in words. Annoying behaviours such as whining, screaming, biting, and temper tantrums subside between two and three years, once the child has enough verbal skills to communicate his needs by words rather than undesirable behaviours. As developmental

skills progress, neediness lessens, at least somewhat. Yet remember, for many children, their needs do not really decrease, they only change. As a child develops, management responsibility shifts: in the early years, you help the child manage her challenging behaviour so that eventually she can manage it herself. In those middle years, you'll spend many hours preparing your child for adult life. And remember, for most high-need children, their brains seem way ahead of their bodies.

Jonathan is now a lovable, cuddly, sensitive, intelligent boy. He always had these qualities; they were just trapped inside the body of a baby. When he learned to walk and talk he became less frustrated with his world, and with our world too. Jim and I now enjoy a life with him that we never thought possible. Our high-need baby has very definitely yielded us a high level of returns.

grandparent). Our youngest daughter, Lauren, was given a videotape when she was about two years and nine months old that included a song entitled "Mama Comes Back." It was her favourite part of the video. She liked Martha to sing the song for her at bedtime over and over. We were still having trouble leaving her happily behind when we went out, and one night we again faced a tearful Lauren who didn't want Martha to leave. Remembering how much Lauren liked this song, Martha suggested that because she was leaving, she'd put on "Mama Comes Back" for her. Her face instantly

brightened and she clicked on to that idea and ran happily to watch the video, secure in the reassurance that Mummy would come back.

the changing personality profile of the high-need child

The words you use to describe your high-need child will change over the years, as the traits that so exhausted you during infancy are channelled into qualities that will make your child an interesting, dynamic adult. Try to think of your child's personality in a positive light and look ahead. Labels that seem like negatives will be positive traits in your child's future personality.

Infant	Toddler-child	Teen-adult
alert	busy	enthusiastic
intense	high-strung	deep
draining	exhausting	passionate
demanding	spunky	resourceful
cries impressively	driven	dominating
loud	energetic	opinionated
inconsolable	stubborn	determined
supersensitive	impatient	persistent
high-touch	strong-willed	discerning
	obstinate	insightful
	challenging	fair
	expressive	sociable
	tantrum-prone	compassionate
	interesting	empathic
	tender	caring
	huggable	affectionate

chapter 3

your baby's cry – what it means, how to listen

At some time during the early months of living with a fussy baby, a well-meaning adviser almost certainly will suggest that you, "let your baby cry it out – he's got to learn sometime". This is misguided advice. It shows not only a misunderstanding of the communication value of the infant's cry, but also a devaluing of the mother's sensitivity.

Mothers are not designed to let their babies cry, nor are babies' cries designed to go unanswered.

"If only my baby could talk instead of cry I would know what she wants", said Jane, a new mother of a fussy baby. "Your baby can talk", we advised. "The key is for you to learn how to listen." Consider how much more aware you have to be when you are in a foreign country struggling to understand someone. You have to pay attention to body language and be more discerning, so that you can use all available clues to figure out what this person is saying. Once you pay attention to the clues, communicating still requires effort, but you quickly get the gist.

A baby's cry ensures the survival of the infant and promotes the development of the parent. It's a two-way communication system designed to get infants whatever they need to thrive, and to teach parents how to interpret their baby's language.

> *But what am I?*
> *An infant crying in the night:*
> *An infant crying for the light:*
> *And with no language but a cry.*
> ALFRED, LORD TENNYSON

When you learn the special language of your baby's cry, you will be able to respond sensitively. Here are some listening tips that will help you discover what your baby is trying to say when he cries.

an infant's cry – the perfect signal

Scientists have long appreciated that the sound of an infant's cry has all four features of a perfect signal. First, a perfect signal is automatic. A newborn cries by reflex. The infant senses a need, which triggers a sudden inspiration of air followed by a forceful expelling of that air through vocal cords, which vibrate to produce the sound we call a cry. In the early months, the tiny infant does not think, "What kind of cry will get me fed?" He just automatically cries. Second, the cry is easily generated. Once his lungs are full of air, the infant can initiate crying with very little effort. Third, the cry is appropriately disturbing: ear-piercing enough to get the caregiver's attention and make him or her try to stop the cry but not so disturbing as to make the listener want to avoid the sound altogether. Fourth, the cry can be modified as both the sender and the listener learn ways to make the signal more precise.

Each baby's signal is unique. A baby's cry is a baby's language, and each baby cries differently. Voice researchers call these unique sounds "cry prints", which are as unique for babies as their fingerprints are.

Once you appreciate the special signal value of your baby's cry, the important thing is what you do about it. You have two basic options: ignore or respond. Ignoring your baby's cry is usually a lose-lose situation. A more compliant baby gives up and stops signalling, becomes withdrawn, eventually realizes that crying is not worthwhile, and concludes that he himself is not worthwhile either. The baby loses the motivation to communicate with his parents, and the parents miss out on opportunities to get to know their baby. Everyone loses. A baby with a more persistent personality does not give up so easily. Instead, he cries more loudly and keeps escalating his signal, making it more and more disturbing. You could ignore this persistent

responding to baby's cries is biologically correct

A mother is biologically programmed to give a nurturant response to her newborn's cries and not to restrain herself. Fascinating biological changes take place in a mother's body in response to her infant's cry. Upon hearing her baby cry, the blood flow to a mother's breasts increases, accompanied by a biological urge to "pick up and feed". The act of breast-feeding itself causes a surge in prolactin, a hormone that we feel forms the biological basis of the term "mother's intuition". Oxytocin, the hormone that causes a mother's milk to let down, brings feelings of relaxation and pleasure, a pleasant release from the tension built up by the baby's cry. These feelings help you love your baby. Mothers, listen to the biological cues of your body when your baby cries rather than to advisers who would tell you to turn a deaf ear. These biological happenings explain why it's easy for those advisers to say such a thing. They are not biologically connected to your baby. Nothing happens to *their* hormones when your baby cries.

signal in several ways. You could wait until the baby stops crying and then pick him up, so that he won't think it was his crying that got your attention. This is actually a type of power struggle; you teach the baby that you're in control, but you also teach him that he has no power to communicate. This shuts down parent-child communication, and in the long run everybody loses.

You could desensitize yourself completely so that you won't be "bothered" at all by the cry; this way you can teach baby he gets responded to only when it's "time". Also, according to this scenario, baby gets used to being in a constant state of want. Not feeling right becomes the norm to be re-created throughout his life. This is another lose-lose situation; baby doesn't get what he needs, and parents remain stuck in a mind-set that doesn't allow them to enjoy the baby's unique personality. Or you could pick baby up to calm him but then put him right back down because "it's not time to feed him yet". He has to learn, after all, to be happy "on his own". Lose-lose again; he will start to cry again and you will feel angry. He will learn that his desires make you angry. And he will learn his communication, though heard, has not been understood, which can lead him to learn to distrust his own perceptions ("Maybe they're right. Maybe I'm not hungry").

Your other option is to give a prompt and nurturant response. This is the win-win way for baby and mother to work out a communication system that helps them both. The mother responds promptly and sensitively so that baby will feel less frantic the next time he needs something. The baby learns to cry "better", in a less disturbing way, since he knows mother will come. Mother structures baby's environment so that there is less need for him to cry; she keeps him close to her if she knows he's tired and ready to sleep. Mother also heightens her sensitivity to the cry so that she can give just the right response: a quick response when the baby is young and prone to fall apart easily or when the cry makes it clear there is real danger, a slower response when the baby is older and can begin to learn to settle the disturbance on his own.

Responding appropriately to your baby's cry is the first and one of the most difficult of many communication challenges you will face as a mother. You will master the system only after rehearsing thousands of cue-response cycles in the early months. If you initially regard your baby's cry as a signal to be responded to and evaluated rather than as an unfortunate habit to be broken, you will open yourself up to becoming an expert in your baby's signals, which will carry over into becoming an expert on everything about your baby. Each mother-baby signal system is unique. That's why it is so short-sighted for "sleep trainers" to prescribe canned cry-response formulas, such as "leave her to cry for five minutes the first night, ten minutes the second", and so on.

should baby cry it out?

"But is there a time when I should leave my baby to cry?" you may wonder. As a new mother you are vulnerable to all kinds of well-meaning advisers, each of whom bears his own bag of tricks to dump on you whether you want them or not. The most damaging of all this free advice is "leave your baby to cry it out". This often given, yet seldom helpful, advice shows a lack of understanding of the signal value of the infant cry and of the receptive qualities of the listening mother. This advice serves no useful purpose; if followed, it usually desensitizes a mother to her baby and creates a distance between the members of the communicating pair.

As a teacher, my training in child development kept haunting me. I remember learning that the social and emotional growth of a child begins with the stage of trust versus mistrust. Jason would either learn trust in his environment or learn various degrees of mistrust. Even if we could not alleviate his discomfort, we could at least hold him and rock him and let him know we cared. Abandoning him to suffer alone in a cot down the hall seemed cruel and inhumane. If we could not comfort him, at least we could teach him to learn to trust.

No one should ever advise a mother to let her baby cry it out, but neither should a mother feel that it is her responsibility always to stop her baby from crying. In the following discussion we want to help you work out the cry-response communication network that works best for you. If, when, and how long to let your baby complain is a cry-by-cry judgment. These following considerations can help you make the right judgement.

How the cry-it-out advice got started. In light of what we now know about infant development,

the cry-it-out advice should be put in its proper place – filed away in the archives of bad baby advice; yet this dreadful advice is still around. Why? Understanding the historical setting that bred this philosophy makes it easier to appreciate why this advice is still so common. This sad story began in the late 1890s, when drastic changes occurred in parenting, ones that, like a contagious disease, are still around infecting parenting practices a hundred years later. This was the era when, due to a variety of social and economic situations, experts entered the business of advising women on childbearing and child rearing. Traditional motherly wisdom fell out of favour and new "scientific" theories took over. Pregnancy and birth became a medical "disease" from which a woman needed to be delivered. Man-made formula replaced mother-made milk. Rigid schedules replaced flexible feeding routines. The infant cry became an annoyance to be squelched, not a signal to be listened and responded to. "What should I do when my baby cries?" was a question that mothers should never have had to ask in the first place, and advisers should not even have attempted to answer.

Once "scientific" notions of baby tending did away with mother's intuition, demand rose in the baby-advice market, and a multitude of advisers rushed in to supply what was needed. The most prevalent parenting theory of the time was that parents must be strict and in control, that babies and children should follow rigid, prescribed routines, and that parents who didn't follow this advice to the letter were likely to raise spoiled and wildly uncontrollable children. If parents listened to their baby rather than to the

survival mode

Even as newborns, most babies who are separated from their mothers click into survival mode: their breathing increases, they clench their fists, they arch their backs and tense their muscles. Their whole body language shouts, "I have to be held to survive." The sooner parents pick up on these cues, the sooner baby will thrive. Some babies are particularly separation-sensitive, even during sleep. We decided to study the physiological effects of nighttime separation on our eighth baby, Lauren, when she was two months old. A local company loaned us £50,000 worth of equipment and their technical assistance. Using the latest in non-invasive technology, we wired Lauren to a computer that recorded her electrocardiogram, breathing movements, air flow from her nose, and her blood oxygen saturation. The instrumentation was painless and didn't appear to disturb her sleep. The computer recorded Lauren's physiological changes during one full night of sleeping side-by-side with Martha and the next full night of sleeping alone in the same bed. Our study revealed that Lauren's overall physiology – her heart rate, breathing, and blood oxygen saturation – was more stable when sleeping next to Martha than when sleeping alone.

New studies are beginning to prove what savvy mothers have long suspected: growing infants develop better the more time they spend in touch and interaction with their parents.

books, they were not in control and their babies were manipulating them. To rescue parents from the fearful prospect of losing control, baby-care advisers handed out quick and easy rules to help parents control their children. The chief vaccine against the disease of manipulation was "let baby cry it out." This was not just a suggestion, it became a mandate. This advice even came with a schedule of the predicted results: baby will probably cry one hour the first night, forty-five minutes the second night, and so on. Every new cry adviser had his own timetable: "Leave baby to cry five minutes before the first time you go in to reassure him, ten minutes the second time …"

How did these parenting "experts" come up with these numbers? One begins to wonder. Wishful thinking? There were no actual studies to back them up. By the time the study of infant behaviour developed into a science in the sixties and seventies and researchers began disproving the spoiling theory, the low-touch, high-control style of parenting was so entrenched that even today compelling research has not been able to unseat it.

The cry-it-out advice is based on the principle of reinforcement, which is simply this: if a behaviour is not reinforced (not responded to), it is extinguished, it goes away. If the behaviour is reinforced (responded to), it will be repeated. This does make a certain amount of sense, but there are several fallacies in the way this principle has been applied to infant crying. First of all, the reinforcement principle assumes that the cry is a bad behaviour to be eliminated rather than a signal to be listened to. Second, research does not support the idea that ignored cries are simply extinguished. Rather than learning to be quiet, some infants learn more disturbing means of communication. In other babies, those with whom the cry-it-out advice "works", it is the drive to communicate that is extinguished. And along with learning that his cries have no signal value, the baby also learns that he has less value. This lays the foundation for a sense of distrust rather than trust. This is no way to begin life.

"But it works", defenders of cry-stopping advice claim. This depends upon your point of view. Consider how you would feel if you had a desperate message to convey, and your previously trusted significant other stopped listening. You're delivering what you feel is a very

---

cry-it-out advice: 1897-style

The following is a quote from one of the most influential baby-care books of the nineteenth century, *Diseases of Infancy and Childhood,* by paediatrician Dr Emmett Holt, published in 1897. This excerpt will help you appreciate the misguided, controlling origins of the cry-it-out advice. After Dr Holt advises mothers to respond to their baby's cries if they believe the cry is due to illness, he goes on to admonish them: "The cry of habit is one of the most difficult to recognize. These habits are formed by indulging infants in various ways. Some children cry to be held, some to be carried, some to be rocked, some for a light in the nursery, some for a rubber nipple or some other thing to suck. The extent to which even very young infants may indulge in this kind of crying, is surprising, and it explains much of the crying of early childhood. The fact that the cry ceases immediately when the child gets what it wants is diagnostic of the cry from habit. The only successful treatment of such cases is to allow the child to 'cry it out' once or twice and then the habit is broken ... On admission to Babies' Hospital very young infants almost invariably cry a great deal for the first two days. It being against the rules to take such children from their cots and hold them to quiet their crying, they soon cease the habit, and give no further trouble ... The mothers were forbidden to quiet the infants by taking them up, and after two or three days' discipline the crying ceased and peace and order were again restored."

Such is the frightening advice that was to infect parenting throughout the next century.

important message, at least to you. You need some help, yet the one to whom you are talking ignores you. How would you feel? You might conclude that what you are saying has little or no value to the listener. You might further conclude that your listener doesn't care about your message, or about you. How would you react? You could yell more loudly and make yourself so obnoxious that your listener would be forced to come to your rescue. By this time you'd be a very angry person and would carry that anger with you, perhaps turning it inward. You could just quit delivering your message, sniffle to yourself a few times, and decide that you can't depend on anyone but yourself or that maybe you don't deserve to be heard. A baby who makes this shift might even be rewarded with the tag of "good baby", one who doesn't bother anyone. A third alternative is to go on delivering your message, sincerely hoping your listeners will stretch themselves to really hear what you have to say, and will respond appropriately.

For some infants, the cry-it-out advice does seem to "work", in that they stop crying as much. These infants seem to be the compliant type, the "easy" babies. And many seem none the worse for wear when trained to become "good babies". The older "easy" baby may wind himself down from a cry, realizing that he can do this without outside help and that he is really all right afterward. This does not happen with high-need babies, as mothers we have interviewed testify. Most of these mothers revealed that if they tried the cry-it-out advice, their babies just kept crying persistently, and afterward both the mothers and their babies were emotional wrecks. In fact, many mothers who have, in desperation, left their babies to cry it out, have later confided, "I'll never do that again."

What cry research tells us. Researchers Sylvia Bell and Mary Ainsworth performed studies in the 1970s that should have put the spoiling theory on the shelf to spoil forever. These researchers studied two groups of mother-infant pairs. Group 1 mothers gave a prompt and nurturant response to their infant's cries. Group 2 mothers were more restrained in their response. They found that children in Group 1 were less likely to use crying as a means of communication at one year of age. These children seemed more securely attached to their mothers and had developed better communicative skills, becoming less whiny and manipulative.

Up until that time parents had been led to believe that if they picked up their baby every time she cried, she would never learn to settle herself and would become more demanding. Bell's and Ainsworth's research showed the opposite. Babies who developed a secure attachment and whose cues were responded to in a prompt and nurturant way became less clingy and demanding. More studies were done to shoot down the spoiling theory, showing that babies whose cries were not promptly responded to began to cry more, longer, and in a more disturbing way. In one study comparing two groups of crying babies, one group of infants received an immediate, nurturant response to their cries, while the other group was left to cry it out. The babies whose cries were sensitively attended to cried 70 per cent less. The babies in the cry-it-out group, on the other hand, did not decrease their crying. In essence, crying research has shown that babies whose cries are listened to and responded to learn to cry "better"; infants who are the product of a more restrained style of parenting learn to cry "harder". It is interesting that the studies revealed differences not only in how the babies communicated with the parents based on the response they got to their cries, but there were also differences in the mothers. Studies showed that mothers who gave a more restrained and less nurturant response gradually became more insensitive to their baby's cries, and this insensitivity carried over to other aspects of their parent-child relationship. Research showed that leaving baby to cry it out spoils the whole family.

Discipline confused with control. Another reason the cry-it-out advice has survived so long is that it was marketed as one of the essential points of discipline. Parents were led to feel that if they didn't let their baby cry they were wimpy parents and that their children would always have the upper hand. This approach to child rearing confused discipline with control, a confusion that persists in some parenting-advice circles. With the parent-in-control philosophy, the infant's temperament and personality play no part in determining the style of care he receives. The infant is given no voice in his own management. This undermines the whole foundation of parental discipline: knowing your infant and creating a trusting relationship between parent and child. Babies, even newborns, can learn the basic principle of trust: distress is followed by comfort, and thus the world of the family is a nurturing and

responsive place to be. In contrast, the cry-it-out advice creates a distance between infants and parents, a distance that makes disciplining the growing child more difficult.

Crying isn't "good for baby's lungs". One of the most ridiculous pieces of medical folklore is the dictum "Let baby cry – it's good for his lungs." In the late 1970s, research showed that babies who were left to cry had heart rates that reached worrisome levels and lowered oxygen levels in their blood. When these infants' cries were soothed, their cardiovascular system rapidly returned to normal, showing how quickly babies recognize the status of well-being on a physiologic level. When a baby's cries are not soothed, he remains in physiological as well as psychological distress.

The erroneous belief about the healthfulness of crying survives even today in one of the items factored into the Apgar score, a test that physicians use to assess a newborn's condition rapidly in the first few minutes after birth. Babies get an extra two points for "crying lustily". I remember pondering this back in the mid-1970s, when I was the director of a university hospital's newborn nursery, even before fathering a high-need baby had turned me into an opponent of crying it out. It seemed to me that awarding points for crying made no sense physiologically. The newborn who was in the state of quiet alertness and breathing normally was actually pinker than a crying infant, even though the quiet baby lost points on the Apgar score. It amazes me that the most intriguing of all human sounds – the infant's cry – is still so misunderstood.

it's not your fault

Parents, take heart! If you are responsive to your baby and try to keep him feeling secure in his new world, you need not feel that it's your fault if your baby cries a lot. Nor is it your job to make your baby stop crying. Of course, you stay open to learning new things to help your baby, like a change in your diet (see Chapter 10), or a new way of wearing baby (see pages 55–6), and you get your doctor involved if you suspect a physical cause behind the crying (see Chapter 10). But there will be times when you won't know why your baby is crying – you'll wonder if baby even knows why he's crying. There may be times when baby needs to cry, perhaps because he just feels stressed. You needn't feel desperate to make him stop after trying all the usual things. It's a fact of new parent life that although babies cry to express a need, the style in which they do so is the result of their own temperament. Don't take your baby's cries personally. Your job is to create a supportive environment that lessens your baby's need to cry, to offer a set of caring and relaxed arms so that your baby does not need to cry alone, and to do as much detective work as you can to figure out why your baby is crying and how you can help. The rest is up to your baby.

When I was confused about my mothering, I asked a seasoned, calm, impartial mother to observe how I handled my baby on a typical day in my home. Even though I know I am the expert on my own baby, sometimes it is hard to be objective, and the voice of experience can be helpful.

Letting baby cry desensitizes mother. Not only is the cry-it-out advice bad for babies, it's bad for mothers. When we began writing about babies, we interviewed hundreds of mothers about their views on the cry-it-out advice. Ninety-five per cent of the mothers told us that this advice went against their basic intuition. It made them feel "not right". We concluded that 95 per cent of mothers couldn't be wrong.

Besides being physiologically harmful to babies, the cry-it-out advice makes no physiologic sense for mothers. The infant's cry affects the mother's body chemistry, and that's what makes it so special. No other sound in the world triggers such intense emotions in the mother. The cry is supposed to do that, and the mother is supposed to feel that way.

Mothers are biologically programmed to respond to their infant's cries. When a mother goes against her basic intuitive response and "hardens her heart against the little tyrant", she desensitizes herself to the language of her infant. This opens the door and lets in the "infection" of insensitivity, which can one day land mother, father, and child in the office of the discipline counsellors. Insensitivity gets new parents into trouble and makes their job more and more difficult.

the shutdown syndrome

Throughout our twenty-five years of working with parents and babies, we have grown to appreciate the correlation between how well children thrive (emotionally and physically) and the style of parenting they receive. First-time parents Linda and Nigel brought their four-month-old high-need baby, Heather, into my surgery for consultation because Heather had stopped growing. Heather had previously been a happy baby, thriving on a full dose of attachment parenting. She was carried many hours a day in a baby sling, her cries were given a prompt and nurturant response, she was breast-fed on cue, and she was literally in physical touch with one of her parents most of the day. The whole family was thriving and this style of parenting was working for them. Well-meaning friends convinced these parents that they were spoiling their baby, that she was manipulating them, and that Heather would grow up to be a clingy, dependent child.

Like many first-time parents, Nigel and Linda lost confidence in what they were doing and yielded to the peer pressure of adopting a more restrained and distant style of parenting. They let Heather cry herself to sleep, scheduled her feedings, and for fear of spoiling, they didn't carry her as much. Over the next two months Heather went from being happy and interactive to sad and withdrawn. Her weight levelled off, and she went from the top of the growth chart to the bottom.

Heather was no longer thriving, and neither were her parents.

After two months of no growth, Heather was labelled by her doctor "failure to thrive" and was about to undergo an extensive medical workup. When the parents consulted me, I diagnosed the shutdown syndrome. I explained that Heather had been thriving because of their responsive style of parenting. Because of their parenting, Heather had trusted that her needs would be met and her overall physiology had been organized. In thinking they were doing the best for their infant, these parents let themselves be persuaded into another style of parenting. They unknowingly pulled the attachment plug on Heather, and the connection that had caused her to thrive was gone. A sort of baby depression resulted, and her physiologic systems slowed down. I advised the parents to return to their previous high-touch, attachment style of parenting: to carry her a lot, breast-feed her on cue, and respond sensitively to her cries by day and night. Within a month Heather was once again thriving.

We believe every baby has a critical level of need for touch and nurturing in order to thrive. (Thriving means not just getting bigger, but growing to one's potential, physically and emotionally.) We believe that babies have the ability to teach their parents what level of parenting they need. It's up to the parents to listen, and it's up to professionals to support the parents' confidence and not undermine it by advising a more distant style of parenting, such as "let your baby cry it out" or "you've got to put him down more." Only the baby knows his or her level of need; and the parents are the ones that are best able to read their baby's language.

Babies who are "trained" not to express their needs may appear to be docile, compliant, or "good" babies. Yet these babies could be depressed babies who are shutting down the expression of their needs, and they may become children who don't ever speak up to get their needs met and eventually become the highest-need adults.

should you *ever* let baby cry?

There cannot be a rigid yes or no answer to this question. The mother-infant communication network is too intricate and sensitive to be subjected to dictums from an outsider. But be warned: it is the rare baby who follows the cry-it-out time charts displayed in various baby books over the past hundred years. These charts promise that crying will diminish; for many babies and in many circumstances this is not true. Nevertheless, there are times when you'd like some guidelines on how to hold up your end of the communication network while still giving your baby opportunities to grow toward independence.

The following guidelines are not meant to override your sensitivity. If, when, and how you decide to let your baby or toddler solve his difficulties without you must remain a parental cry-by-cry judgement.

Here are some suggestions to help you decide how quickly you need to respond to cries:

1. **Listen to yourself.** Listen to your own inner sensitivity as to whether any part of the cry-it-out approach is right for you, right for your baby, right for your baby's stage of development, or right for your individual family circumstances – regardless of the norms of your friends.

2. **Consider the depth of your attachment with your baby.** If you practise the overall style of attachment parenting, are a high-touch, high-response parent, and have a healthy trust relationship with your baby, then you can become more restrained in your cry response without damaging that trust as baby grows older. In fact, your knowledge of your baby will help you here. You'll know which cries need an immediate response and which ones are the sounds of your baby working things out on her own. You'll respond instantly to the cry of a ten-*day*-old baby, be able to discern what's wrong when a ten-*week*-old cries, while still responding quickly, and when a ten-*month*-old cries, your discernment may lead you to delay your response for a few minutes.

3. **Use baby as the barometer.** Don't lock yourself into a set number of minutes or nights

that you will delay your response to your baby's cry. Let baby's overall behaviour influence your decision as to whether or not your response time is right for you and your baby. Don't persist with a bad experiment.

4. **Consider your baby's temperament.** Easier-temperament babies are more likely to resettle without your help. The intensity of their cries gradually winds down as they learn to self-soothe. Not so the high-need baby, whose cries continue to escalate.

5. **Analyse whether you are reinforcing baby's cry.** The closer you and your baby are, the more you may, without realizing it, be giving your baby a message that "you need to cry". Mothers mirror emotions to their babies. If you are anxious, baby perceives that there really is something to cry about. I see this often in my paediatric practice. Parents new to our practice bring their infant into the surgery for a check-up. Seeing a stranger, baby begins to fuss and clings to mum. This makes mum anxious and she clings back to baby, giving baby the message that there really is something to be afraid about.

Let's replay this scenario. Suppose this mother puts on her best everything's-okay face, giving baby the message that she is calm and in control. Then, if baby fusses, she continues her, "it's okay" body language, while at the same time reassuring baby with a cool "it's no big deal" attitude. A certain amount of anxiety is appropriate in strange situations, but it's up to mum to model the calm behaviour she wants her baby to learn.

I have noticed that first-time parents sometimes panic at their baby's cries and jump every time their baby makes a peep. Veteran parents, on the other hand, are better able to distinguish "biggies", those cries needing prompt attention, from "smallies", those triggered by something baby can handle with little or no help, or they have learned to meet baby's needs before baby has to cry. (See related discussions "Don't Panic!" opposite, and "No Problem", page 72.)

6. **Consider how important your need to let baby self-settle is.** One of the most difficult parts of parenting is weighing baby's needs against your needs, for example, your need for sleep versus baby's need to be comforted. Signals that your parental balance system needs adjustments include these: You are not enjoying motherhood; you are having second thoughts about the style of parenting you are doing; you are becoming a tired and cranky mother, and the whole family is suffering. One of the principles that we have found helpful in our own family and in counselling other mothers who are burning out is this one:

if you resent it, change it

If you are beginning to resent your style of parenting and your constant baby tending and are feeling at the mercy of your baby's cries, take this as a signal that you need to make a change somewhere in your cry-response system. This is more easily said than done and may not necessarily mean that crying it out is the solution. In the following section and in the chapters to come we will help you find ways to

don't panic!

Patricia, a new mother of a high-need baby, was a psychologist specializing in child development. Because clients with low self-esteem had consumed her counselling days, she was determined that she would bring up her child to have healthy self-esteem. She understood the value of giving a nurturant response to her baby's cries. But baby Christopher didn't just cry, he shrieked. Within the first millisecond of Christopher's shriek, Patricia would jump up, a tense mother with a worried face, inadvertently increasing his tension and sending him into an all-out fit that could have been avoided.

Martha watched this behaviour unfold one day when Patricia was over for a visit. Patricia had come over for Martha's advice because she couldn't get Christopher to go into the sling. Each time she tried, Christopher would shriek, and Patricia would panic and quickly end the lesson by grabbing her baby out of the sling and calming him. Martha showed Patricia several ways of positioning Christopher in the sling, and, sure enough, each position was unpopular with Christopher. Patricia would visibly tense up and look worried until Martha suggested another position. Finally, Martha figured out which position worked best for the two of them, and then, although Christopher was beginning to fret, Martha calmly said, "Now let's go for a walk around the block." This had two results. Christopher started to relax as Patricia started moving, and Patricia took her mind off the baby for a few minutes.

Martha and Patricia chatted as they walked, and Christopher became more and more relaxed. Soon Patricia was sensing that Christopher was actually enjoying the sling, and they both relaxed even more, so much so that the baby fell asleep. Patricia learned that she could mirror relaxation to her baby by staying calm and walking onward despite the fussing. Christopher needed his mother to set the mood and allow him enough time to follow suit. Patricia discovered that without much effort her baby would catch mum's mood, and they could relax together.

Don't let yourself panic at baby's first squeak. This overreaction relays the message to baby that there really is something to fuss about, and he will usually oblige. For some babies, the quick response will ward off a hysterical cry; for others, it stimulates it. This is why you have to play each cry by ear. As soon as your baby starts to fuss, put on a relaxed "it's okay" expression as you calmly tend to him. With a baby of four or five months, you can delay your response a minute or so, depending on the time of day and the situation, to see if baby discovers on his own that there is nothing to fuss about. Throughout the day, each episode will need an individual response. I notice a difference between many first-time mothers, who get easily panicked by the first whimper and are hyper-responsive, and seasoned veterans, who take a more relaxed, but still nurturant, approach to responding to baby's crying.

meet both your needs and those of your baby and provide sensitive practical alternatives.

Giving the right response for each situation is part of being mature as a parent. And guess what? You don't always have to get it right. Babies are forgiving, and they seem to appreciate that at least you are trying. It's not your fault that your baby cries; nor is it always your responsibility to keep baby from crying. Your job is to set the conditions to lessen baby's need to cry and to offer a nurturant response when baby does need to cry. The rest is up to baby.

mellowing baby's cries

All babies cry, but some cries are easier to tolerate and respond to than others. Here are some practical things you can do with your baby to mellow her cries from mind-shattering screams to easy-listening communication.

Start early. When I was director of a newborn nursery, I learned a lot from veteran nurses who had spent years coping with crying babies. There wasn't a sound they hadn't heard and learned to live with. These nurses used to tag the babies' temperaments as early as the first day of life: "Jason's going to be easy", or "Susannah's going to be a handful", or "George's cry is going to shatter his mother's nerves." I realized the importance of mellowing a baby's cry early on so that it can promote mother-infant attachment instead of mother-infant avoidance.

Baby Charlie was the second-born child of an easygoing and nurturing mother. During her pregnancy Janine would tell me, "I can tell this baby's going to be a challenge by the way he kicks. He's been a tummy-pounder and a bladder-thumper all during my pregnancy." Her prediction came true. Charlie came out crying, and kept crying. He announced to the world that his was a voice to be reckoned with. Even during that magnificent passage from obstetrician's hands to mother's breasts Charlie let out a shriek that startled the obstetrician so much that Janine feared he would drop him. While most newborn's cries evoke a sympathetic and tender feeling in the listener, Charlie's did not. His cries were so shrill, they made everyone want to plug their ears and run. Charlie's cries soon cleared the birth room.

Janine, an otherwise unflappable mother, cringed when her baby shrieked. The nursery nurses couldn't stand Charlie's quickly escalating cries, so at the first shriek they would immediately shuttle him out to his mother (which was good for Charlie, who wanted to be with his mother).

On the day of discharge, Janine confided to me that Charlie's cries were interfering with her relationship with her baby. She admitted she didn't have those love-at-first-sight feelings new mothers are supposed to have. I knew that many infants' cries become steadily more shrill and disturbing at two weeks of age than when they are newly born. If we didn't do something, Charlie's cries – and his relationship with his family – were going to get worse instead of better.

So Janine and I developed a three-part plan to help mellow out Charlie's cries. My instructions to her were as follows:

1. Wear him almost constantly in the baby sling so he has no need to fuss about feeling alone.
2. Feed him frequently, at least every two hours during the day, and as needed during the night. Don't wait for him to fuss to announce feeding time. As soon as he opens his mouth for anything more than a yawn, fill it with a breast within the first millisecond. (Jan knew I was exaggerating, but she got the point.)
3. Keep a list of situations that set off Charlie's cries. Try to anticipate his needs and feed him, rock him, sing to him – whatever it takes to keep him from crying.

I also suggested Charlie's parents tape-record his cries so they could keep track of their progress in mellowing Charlie's temperament. Sure enough, within a week Janine said, "I finally enjoy being with him. He cries much nicer now."

Why do some infants cry with such shrill, nerve-racking noises? Having seen several babies like this one who were "born" criers, I have come to wonder if the baby is affected by the stress hormones that mother made in order to handle a particularly stressful pregnancy or painful delivery.

Give baby a calm start. Some babies are born criers, but the care they get during the first few days can influence whether or not they stay that way. Let's look at the two room-accommodation options a newborn used to have: a slot in the nursery or a spot close to mum.

The nursery option. Fresh from a soft, warm womb and a little time in mother's arms, a baby born even relatively recently would take a bumpy ride to the newborn nursery, where he would stay on a static mattress in a plastic box, surrounded by bright lights, chatty adults, and a line-up of other babies in plastic boxes. What he needed was to stay with his mother so that he could gaze at her face and use her smell, her movements, and her holding to help him stay calm and feel safe. He was miserable and frightened in the plastic box and cried desperately. If there was a nurse there who had time, she might pick him up, but chances are he'd have to wait. He'd cry and cry until he exhausted himself to sleep, in the process experiencing very disturbing feelings. Bonding was severely disrupted, and he learnt that he could not trust that his needs would be met.

The nursery option was a biologically incorrect set-up. The nurse was the one who initially heard the baby's cry, but the mother (in another room) is the one who is biologically programmed to calm the cries. Most infants have two phases to their cry. The early phase, called the attachment-promoting phase, is the perfect signal, disturbing enough to prompt the listener to want to pick up and hold the baby and give a comforting response, but not so disturbing as to make the listener want to avoid the baby. In the nursery arrangement, this is the phase of the cry that the nurse heard, and she eventually took the baby down to the mother's room. However, by the time baby got to his mother, his cries were in the next phase – the avoidance-promoting phase. His cries escalate into a shrill sound, and the mother is presented with an anxious, frightened baby whose cries cause her to be anxious, even frightened. The mother is the one person who is biologically programmed to calm the cries,

know your limits

Nothing pierces parents' hearts more than the cry of their baby. Yet cries can push dangerous buttons, too: feelings of anger, helplessness, despair – feelings that may overwhelm you and fill your mind with scary thoughts. Some very loving mothers have confided to us crazy thoughts they've had, such as throwing their baby out the window. And while it's not unusual to plead with your baby to "please, be quiet", there are good mothers who, on occasion, actually scream "shut up" at their baby. These feelings are aggravated even more by the fatigue that comes with parenting a fussy baby.

You can guard against doing something that you would immediately regret by rehearsing ahead of time what you would do if you felt yourself about to snap. Programme this behaviour into your mind, play-act it when things are going well, so that you will know how to react if you are pushed past your limit. When you feel overwhelmed by anger, feel like yelling at your baby, or feel that you are at your wit's end, do one of the following: hand your baby to a less distressed set of arms; put your baby down momentarily and walk out of the room to compose yourself; put your baby in the sling and take a long, hard walk; or call an empathic friend, one who has survived the same trials.

Having these angry feelings does not mean that you are not a good mother. The mothers most bothered by their infant's cries are often the ones who are most sensitive. Sensitivity can work to your advantage as a mother because it prompts you to try many ways of comforting your baby. Yet this same sensitivity can also set you up to feel like a failure if you can't stop the crying. Having these feelings means that you are a tired mother, and your baby's cries are getting to you. Take these emotions as a signal that you need some help in managing your feelings, managing your own care, and managing your baby's cries.

yet she is not present for the opening sounds that would have made this an easy, welcome job. Mothers and babies who started out life in separate rooms were out of sync. In fact, studies have shown that infants who show long bouts of anxious and disturbing crying (dubbed the "infant distress syndrome") were placed in the nursery rather than kept with mother from birth.

The rooming-in option. Baby awakens in mother's arms or with mother nearby and begins to cry. Because mother is right there, she hears the attachment-promoting sounds of baby's cry, which trigger in her a nurturant response. She immediately caresses and comforts her baby – before the cry has to escalate into a more disturbing sound or enter the avoidance-promoting phase. After several of these cry-response rehearsals, mother learns to recognize baby's pre-cry cues: a squirm, a grimace, followed by lip-smacking attempts to find something to suck on. Mother offers her breast before baby has to cry. Soon baby learns that he does not have to cry, certainly not in a disturbing way, to get what he needs. (As an added perk, the attachment-promoting phase of the infant's cry can trigger the release of mother's milk-releasing hormones, giving her a biologic boost for comforting; the avoidance-promoting phase of the infant's cry can tie the mother up in knots, inhibiting her milk-releasing reflex.)

Early in my years as a newborn nursery director, I realized the difference between how nursery-reared and rooming-in babies act. We used to say, "Nursery-reared babies learn to cry *harder*, rooming-in babies learn to cry *better*."

Imagining how your newly born baby feels can be a learning experience for a new mother who is struggling to develop a parenting style. *Everything* changes for the baby at birth. Think how he must feel in the drastically new environment in which he finds himself. He goes from warm, dark, smooth wetness, where he is held on all sides, and never experiences need of any kind, to cold, light, rough dryness, where he is alarmingly free on all sides and experiences a desperate need to be securely held. He has never felt the sensation of hunger before, and initially does not know that mother will ease it for him. He only knows that if he can suck he will survive. This terrifying hunger thing must be stopped! It is crucial that mother be there before baby becomes anxious and frantic (and this is possible only if they are not in separate rooms). Then baby learns not to associate the feeling of

why babies in other cultures cry less

Infant-care specialists who study parenting styles around the world have noticed that infants in more "primitive" cultures usually cry less. One of the reasons for this diminished crying is that infants in these cultures spend most of their day in someone's arms. Unlike babies in Western cultures, who spend much of their time in cots or infant seats, babies in many other cultures are carried in the caregiver's arms or in a sling. In fact, some cultures have a "ground-touching ceremony". Around six months of age babies are ceremoniously put down to crawl on the ground, and they do so quite happily. Mothers continue to hold and carry children as often as the children want, up to three years of age. Western cultures are finally catching on to what other cultures have long known – carried babies cry less.

Dr Melvin Konner, a physician and anthropologist who studies infant-care practices around the world, once translated a fear-of-spoiling passage from a best-selling American infant-care book to a group of African parents in a primitive tribe who practise a high-touch, attachment style of parenting, and whose infants are noted for their calmness. After hearing the warning about spoiling babies from picking them up too often, these mothers responded, "Doesn't he [the author] understand it's only a baby, that's why it cries? You pick it up. Later when it's older, it will have sense. It won't cry anymore." In essence, these intuitive parents rejected the spoiling theory as utter nonsense.

hunger with the feeling of distress. This realization is one of the earliest "house rules" that baby can learn: crying frantically when hungry is neither necessary nor the norm in this strange new life.

Mellow out yourself. One of the most difficult things about parenting for a novice mother is keeping her cool when baby loses his. It's a perfectly normal reaction for a new mother, on the first note of her baby's cry, to jump up immediately, rush to the baby, pick her up with tense arms, stare at baby intently as if to say "What's wrong?!", and begin frantically bouncing baby up and down as if trying to jiggle the cry out of him. It's as though the mother is reacting out of guilt and fear that something she did – putting the baby down alone perhaps – caused the crying. Even though she means this tense reaction as a loving gesture of comfort, the baby may catch her worry, and the cry will escalate. A more effective reaction would start with putting on her best worry-free face, calmly and smoothly picking baby up to comfort him, and rocking in an easy, slow motion, giving baby the message "I'm right here. I won't put you down again."

Though some new mothers are more anxious than others, they can all learn the easy art of baby calming. Having confidence in your

crying and child abuse

One day I was counselling a teenage mother who had confessed to beating her one-year-old child with a wooden spoon. During our session, this usually capable and caring girl broke down crying. "His cries were so grating on my nerves, and he wouldn't stop. Those shrieks just got to me, and I got so angry. I had flashbacks of my father hitting me with a wooden spoon during one of my tantrums. Before I knew it, I grabbed the wooden spoon and let this poor little baby have it."

Child abuse studies have shown the following findings:

- Battered babies generally have more disturbing cries.
- Battering parents are more likely to label their babies "difficult".
- Battering parents are more likely to practise a less responsive style of parenting.

It is important to teach babies to cry, "better", so they don't develop an ear-grating cry that triggers anger rather than empathy. Much child abuse could be avoided by teaching parents who are at risk for child abuse (families in high-stress situations and parents who were themselves abused as children) to give a nurturant response to their baby's cries. The prevention of child abuse is another example of the good that can happen when parents learn to listen to their babies.

mothering skills is the first step. You will notice that an experienced mother can often comfort your baby more easily than you can, at least temporarily. Watch her perform. The baby's cry doesn't rattle her; but slowly, calmly, in a relaxed, yet caring way, she uses her whole body to give the baby the message that there is no need to cry harder. She transmits her quiet confidence to the baby, and the baby incorporates her relaxed attitude into his own state of being. Even if you're new to mothering, you can still feel confident. From the moment your baby is born, you are the person who knows him best. Trust yourself.

Anticipate. The best way to ward off an all-out wail is to try, as much as possible, to set conditions so that baby does not have to cry to get her needs met. Try to read your baby's pre-cry signals and intervene at that point; don't let her learn that she has to cry loudly to get a response. The skill of anticipating cries can come only after days and weeks of baby watching, learning to pick up on little cues that say that your baby needs something, that a cry is soon to follow. If your baby sucks on her fingers, seems disappointed, and then starts to cry, next time feed her when the finger sucking begins, a cue that she is hungry. You'll avoid the crying stage. Developing your skills as a baby-comforter means walking that fine line between responding too quickly and waiting too long. This will be different for different babies and in different situations. Don't worry, your baby will grade you mainly on your effort, not on whether you always read the cues right.

danger zone

The feeling that you want to shake your baby is a red flag, signalling a need for immediate help. Sometimes the ear-shattering shrieks of a hurting, colicky baby can stretch a parent to the point of irrational anger when the parent just wants to "shake it out of him". Angrily shaking baby's fragile brain and spinal structures can cause permanent, sometimes fatal, damage. Cry-sis (now called Serene) operates a hotline for parents to call if they feel themselves reaching this point. 020 7474 5011.

Show baby a sweeter sound. Give baby a sound he likes to hear better than his own cry. Crying quickly becomes self-perpetuating – the more loudly baby cries, the more he is driven to cry. By interrupting a cry long enough to get eye contact you can help him stop. To calm a high-need baby you need to come up with a wide repertoire of sounds. As soon as your infant starts crying, begin humming, singing, whistling, talking nonsense, whatever loud or soft voice or facial contortion catches your baby's attention mid-cry and prompts him to listen to you. Gesturing and whispering "Shhhh" is unlikely to mute a melodramatic crier. Yet this "shush" sound repeated rhythmically over and over resembles the sound of uterine blood flow and, once you get baby's attention, may be a familiar sound that soothes.

Don't expect competing sounds to mellow your baby's cry every time, but it is good practice to get an early start teaching baby which sounds trigger pleasant responses. Crying babies often turn into whiny toddlers, and you can call on the ear-pleasing sounds learned in babyhood to improve the audio quality of the toddler's communication. Give your toddler the message "I don't respond to whining" by telling him, "Let mummy hear your big boy voice, and then we'll go out and play." The earlier you begin practising these voice lessons, the more likely they are to work.

chapter 4

creative ways to soothe a fussy baby

Babies fuss and parents comfort. That's a realistic fact of new family life. Developing your skills as a baby-comforter will be your first priority as a new parent. If you include feeding and changing baby's nappy on the list of comforting interactions with your new baby, keeping your baby comfortable will occupy almost every waking minute you spend together.

Comforting a fussy baby can be as easy as taking an afternoon walk around the room or as hard as climbing a mountain at 2am. While many people intuitively do the right things to calm a fussy baby (probably because these things were done for them), others are thrown into a panic and don't have a clue (probably because they were not comforted as infants).

It helps to understand what calms a baby and why. Most calming techniques involve at least one of these four things:

- rhythmic motion
- soothing sounds
- visual delights and distractions
- close physical contact and touching

Most calming techniques (except visual ones) are like re-creating the womb baby has been used to for nine months. This chapter contains baby-calming techniques that worked with our own fussy babies or that we have learned from experienced baby-calmers in our paediatric practice. Remember, your baby has individual needs. Try these techniques as a starting point, and improvise. After a few months, you and your baby will have a large repertoire of fuss-busters that work.

motions that mellow

1. Wearing Baby in a Sling

A baby carrier will be your most useful fuss-preventing tool. Infant-development researchers who study baby-care practices are

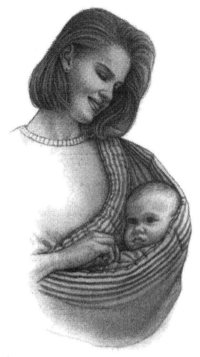

Babywearing.

unanimous in reporting infants who are carried more cry less. In fact, research has shown that babies who are carried at least three hours a day cry 40 per cent less than infants who aren't carried as much. Over the years in paediatric practice, I have listened to and watched veteran baby-calmers and heard a recurrent theme: "As long as I have my baby in my arms or on my body, she's content." This observation led us to popularize the term "babywearing". "Wearing" means more than just picking up baby and putting him in a carrier when he fusses. It means carrying baby many hours a day before baby needs to fuss. This means the carrier you choose must be easy to use and versatile. We have found the sling-type carrier to be the most conducive

to baby-wearing. Baby becomes like part of your apparel and you can easily wear your baby in a sling many hours a day. Mothers who do this tell us, "My baby seems to forget to fuss." The sling is not only helpful for high-need babies, it's essential. Here's why babywearing works.

The outside womb. Being nestled in the arms, against the chest, and near the parent's face gives baby the most soothing of all environments. Mother's walking motion "reminds" baby of the rhythm he enjoyed while in the womb. The sling encircles and contains the infant who would otherwise become agitated and waste energy flinging arms and legs around. The worn baby is only a breath away from the parent's voice, the familiar sound he has grown to associate with feeling good. Babies settle better in this "live" environment than they do when parked in swings or plastic infant seats.

Sights aplenty. Being up in arms gives baby a visual advantage. He now has a wider view of his world. Up near adult eye level, there are more visual attractions to distract baby from fussing.

sucking to soothe

Since babies start sucking while in the womb, they are born relating sucking to soothing. That is one reason why they are so eager to suck right after birth, whether they find a breast or their hands. They need soothing after their wild ride down the birth canal. Mothers intuitively offer sucking to a fussy baby, and it usually works like a charm.

The distressed infant can now pick from a wide array of ever-changing scenery, select what delights him, and shut out what disturbs him. And seen from such a secure perch, even the disturbing sights soon become interesting rather than frightening. You don't have to focus on bringing artificial sights to baby's face. Just your going about your business and varying your movements and environment as you do is enough stimulation for most babies.

Instant replay. The expanding mind of a growing infant is like a video library containing thousands of tapes. These tapes record behaviour patterns that baby has learned to anticipate as either soothing or disturbing. Babywearing mothers tell us, "As soon as I put on the sling, my baby's face lights up with delight, and he stops fussing." The scene of mother putting on the sling triggers a replay in baby's mind of all the pleasant moments she's experienced in mother's arms, and she can anticipate the pleasant interaction that is soon to follow. She stops fussing. She's no longer bored.

Makes life easier for parents. Not only is babywearing good for the infant, it's good for the mother as well. The carrier gives you a comforting tool that usually works. After baby gets used to being worn and you get used to wearing baby, you have more options and more mobility. You'll feel as though you've gained an extra pair of hands, especially around the house, and you can go more places. Baby is content, since "home" to a tiny baby is being with mum, even though mum may be in the middle of a busy shopping centre or at a party full of adults.

A baby who fusses less is more fun to be with and drains less energy from the parents. Infants and parents can then direct the energy they would have wasted on managing fussing into growing and interacting. That's why carried babies thrive – as do their parents.

Familiarity breeds content. Living in a carrier keeps infants content because it keeps them in constant contact with the familiar sounds, touches, movements, and visual delights of their parents. Being nestled in a familiar position is especially calming for the baby who is easily distracted and falls apart at the first sight of a strange person or a strange place. The worn baby is always surrounded by things he knows. From this secure base, the baby has less fear of the unfamiliar – and adjusts without a fuss.

Proximity fosters calmness. A baby who is worn is in mother's arms and literally right under her face. With this close proximity, mother can teach baby to cry "better". As soon as baby gives a hint that he is about to fuss, mother, because she is right there, can pre-empt the cry or keep it from escalating into an all-out fit. Being close to your baby helps you learn to read your baby's pre-cry signals so that you can intervene to meet baby's needs before he has to fuss. Baby in turn learns to be more at ease using non-crying modes of signalling since, during baby-wearing, he has learned that these signals receive an immediate nurturing response.

Sling time for stress time. Once each of our sling babies (Matthew, Stephen, and Lauren) was past the "fussy toddler hanging on to mum's leg" stage, we would pack up our slings, thankful that he or she had matured out of needing to be carried around for long stretches of time. However, we kept one sling handy for those times, even at two and a half or three years, when a certain type of misbehaviour would signal us that instead of "time out" what was needed was "time in". Time in the sling could transform a stressed child into one who would be back to playing pleasantly in ten minutes. Legs were a bit longer, but the little one would snuggle gratefully into the once-familiar position on Martha's hip. Somehow finding that this place was still available seemed to be all the child needed to get back on an even keel. And Martha was grateful that she could comfort a distressed child with relatively little effort.

Babywearing and daycare. Carrie had a high-need baby who was content as long as she was in a sling, but Carrie had to return to work when Mary was six weeks of age. I wrote the following "prescription" to give to her daycare provider:

WILLIAM SEARS M.D.

NAME *Baby Mary*
To keep baby content, wear baby in a sling at least 3 hours a day.
REFILLS *as needed*
Wm. P. Sears, M.D.

How to wear your baby in a sling. Some mothers take to babywearing like a duck takes to water; others may initially find the sling awkward. Also, some babies at first have difficulty settling in the sling. Perhaps they find it too confining. For the best long-term results, get your baby used to being worn in the first week, so that she soon realizes that the sling is where she belongs. It takes some practice, but the sling will soon become your norm of infant care. Take lessons from veteran parents who have logged many miles wearing their babies in a sling in various carrying positions and in many circumstances. Find one of these experts to show you how to wear the sling so it's most comfortable for you and most settling for baby. Keep experimenting with various positions until you find one that works; the favourite position may change with baby's moods and motor development. Most high-need babies prefer to be carried in the forward-facing position (see figure opposite).

For a busy parent of a fussy infant, a baby sling will be one of your most indispensable infant-care items. You won't get dressed without it.

I thought I would definitely have a baby who slept through the night, in his cot, in his room, and that he would awake only to feed and for nappy changes. How naive! Jason knew what kind of parenting he needed right from the start. He was truly a fussy baby, and we nicknamed him "More". He screamed if I put him down even to get dressed. He seemed to nurse constantly, and he rarely slept. As long as he was in my arms or nestled on my husband's chest, he was content,

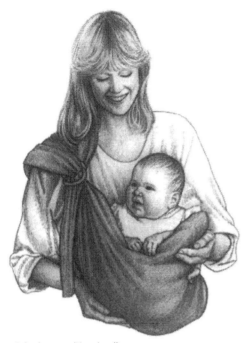

Forward-facing position in sling.

happy, and alert. Any deviation from that was a disaster for everyone. A friend of mine recommended a baby sling so that I could have my hands free to do other things and not begin to feel resentful of all the time a baby takes up. The sling was our saviour! I loved carrying him, and it allowed me to get other things done. The sling ended the pass-the-baby-around sport that so many parents have accepted as just the way things are. There is no way Jason would have stood for being bounced around from person to person for an entire day. An added benefit of the sling was that he was able to feed anywhere and everywhere while in the sling. We went everywhere with him – weddings, funerals, dinners, grocery shopping, doctor visits, vacations, everywhere. Christmas shopping with

Jason in the sling was a breeze. I can't imagine how mothers can manoeuvre buggies through the narrow aisles in most shops. Everywhere we went people remarked how wonderful my baby was. I always pointed out that since my child felt right and was getting his needs met, he really had no reason to be upset.

We observe lots of babywearing pairs in our surgery and at parenting conferences. We're always struck by the fact that we seldom see a sling baby cry.

2. Dancing with Your Baby

Watch a room full of veteran baby-calmers and you will witness a wide variety of dance steps. Each parent has found the dance routine that best suits the mood of both partners, adult and infant. In fact, you can usually spot mothers of high-need babies in a crowd – even without their babies. They are the ones who are swaying back and forth all the time. A mother once told me that as she was standing at a party holding a glass of ginger ale, another mother came up and commented on the fact that she seemed to be

sucking on the move

Sometimes motion alone won't calm a frantic baby; she needs an additional relaxation inducer. Settle baby in a sling-type carrier and, while walking or dancing, offer baby the breast, bottle, or a finger to suck on. Motion and sucking are a winning combination that settles even the most upset baby.

making baby-dancing fun

In baby-dancing, style is as important as getting the steps right. Here are some tips that can make dancing with your baby more comforting and more fun.

Hold your partner
Cling to your little partner in whatever position works. Try the neck nestles, warm fuzzy, colic carries, arm drapes, forward-facing hold, elbow rest, hip carry, or shoulder ride (see figures, pages 67–9). During the first three to four months, be sure to support your partner's wobbly head.

Choose the right rhythm
How fast to dance? Remember, while in the womb your baby was used to the rhythm of your pulse, usually around sixty to seventy beats per minute. Try to rock and swing to this rhythm, approximately one beat per second – "one and a two and a …" The volume, tempo, and type of music may change with your baby's mood and your own. Baby's womb environment is actually quite noisy, so don't be surprised if your baby prefers "big band" sounds.

Choose light dancing
Select a dance that you like, one that suits your mood and energy level, lest the dancer wear out before the fusser. One rainy night Lauren could not give herself up to sleep. Martha racked her brain for what to do next,

when inspiration came from the weather. She started singing "Raindrops Keep Falling on My Head" and did a very jazzy dance step to match the jazzy tune. Lauren soon forgot she was resisting, relaxed into the fun, and nodded off before long. This winning tune got replayed and danced to for many a night thereafter. Martha looked forward to it as a fun way to lull Lauren into Dreamland.

Use props
To keep your arms from wearing out before your legs do, nestle baby in a sling as you dance.

Dinner dance
Some babies love to breast-feed in the sling while you dance. Your movement plus baby's sucking is a winning combination for settling even the most upset baby.

Change partners
Babies usually prefer dancing with mother; after all, she's the dance partner baby came to know even before birth. It's as if baby says to the mother, "I like your style." This also explains why some fathers get frustrated when they try to cut in, offering some relief to worn-out dancer mum. Sometimes babies vehemently protest this change in partners, and father hands baby back to mother saying, "You take her, I give up." Yet many

high-need babies like a change in routine and welcome dad's different holds and steps. And don't forget to invite grandmother to the dance. She has patient and experienced arms and can probably show baby some pretty fancy stepping from her days as a baby-dancer.

teetering back and forth a bit. The observer concluded, "I know you haven't had too much to drink. You must have a baby!"

It's only natural that movement calms fussy babies. Their whole uterine existence was a moving experience. Babies crave movement after birth because to them it is the norm. Being still disconcerts babies. They don't understand it and it frightens them. Movement relaxes them.

One of our hobbies as a couple is ballroom dancing, so this way of relaxing our babies, and ourselves, came naturally. Babycalming by dancing is based on the physiologic principle called "vestibular stimulation". There are three tiny balances that make up the vestibular system, located behind baby's ear. These are set for three planes of movement: up and down, back and forth, and side to side. Dance steps that use all three of these movements stimulate the vestibular system best and are most likely to comfort baby. If babies could choreograph their own dance steps, the routines that contain movements in all three planes would be their favourites. Here are the dance routines that worked best for us. Try these, but remember that the key to baby-dancing is *improvising*.

The swing. Hold your partner in the neck nestle or teddy bear snuggle position (see pages 69 and 75) and sway from side to side with as much movement as baby likes. This side-to-side swaying motion is the most natural dance step for parents.

The dip. This step is a variation of the swing. Bend your knees and then in **a** swaying motion come back up slowly and repeat the motion.

The hop. This hop is the kind you do by bending your knees as you lift first one foot off the floor slightly, then the other foot. You do a hopping motion on the foot that's bearing your weight. (Your feet don't leave the ground at the same time.) Count "one-two" (left foot) then "three-four" (right foot) as you alternate. Sway from side to side as you alternate feet. To put more bounce in your hop, come up on your toes if baby likes that.

The bounce. Hold baby face-to-face with one hand under her bottom and the other supporting her neck. Bounce gently up and down at a rate of sixty to seventy beats per minute using your arms and/or legs. Look at the baby and make eye contact. Another variation is to place baby in this dance hold and bounce gently on a trampoline or while sitting on a physio ball. Some babies like to bounce more vigorously than others, so experiment. Often the higher the need, the harder the bounce. The

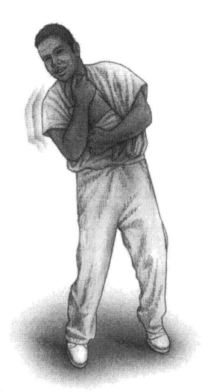

The swing.

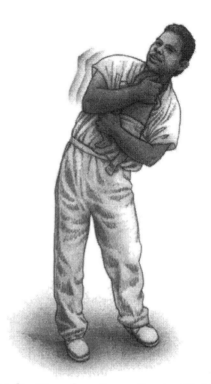

baby needs you to match her energy level. But be wary of using too much force. This dance should never be an excuse to punish the baby. If baby's cries continue as you bounce harder, you could find yourself growing angry and bouncing hard enough to hurt baby. This would be like shaking baby (see page 53). Stop bouncing, cool down, and try something else.

The rock. This is a simple back-and-forth movement as you bend at the waist (and knees, too, if you have the energy). Once you've got the hang of this, you can coordinate this motion with swaying from side to side.

The waltz. One of our favourites (and babies' too), this step is simply a slide and glide movement as you go up on the toe of one foot, then glide the other foot forward to meet it. If you've never learned to waltz, you might want to add some music to help you get the rhythm. A simplified up-and-down version that you can do by taking exaggerated steps while walking we have dubbed the "elevator step". Add some sways and dips and you have movement in all three planes of the baby's vestibular system.

The tango. Most babies prefer smooth dances, but for some fussy infants the abrupt stops, starts, and changes in direction of the tango catch them by surprise and distract them from fussing.

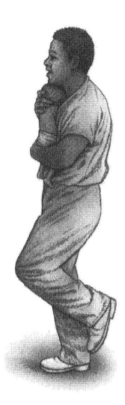

The hop.

The twirl. While most of your dances will be in the three calming directions of up and down, back and forth, and side to side, some babies appreciate the addition of a twirl to your dance routine. Hold baby in the bounce position. Twirl 180 degrees and come to an abrupt stop. A baby who is in full wail usually has his eyes squeezed shut. This abrupt stop will cause him to open his eyes. If you can make eye contact with him right away and keep moving, he'll probably abandon his wailing and watch you, at least momentarily.

3. Swinging Baby

Walk past any playground or peer into any nursery and you'll see happy babies swinging contentedly. The regular swinging motion calms babies. To meet the high demands of fussy babies and frantic parents, infant-product manufacturers have introduced a variety of baby swings to the ever-growing market of baby-soothing devices. None of these synthetic substitutes works as well as the encircling arms, soft breasts, or warm body of a parent, all of which remind baby of the womb. But let's face it, substitute arms are sometimes necessary to save a parent's sanity or at least allow mother to take a shower.

Swings are particularly useful during "happy hour", that stretch of time in the late afternoon to early evening when you're busy preparing or having dinner and babies are notoriously

be comfortable

In building your personal repertoire of baby-calmers, practise mainly the soothing techniques that you like. Chances are that baby will like them too. High-need babies are highly perceptive (of course). They can usually tell when you are using a fuss-buster you really don't like but feel obligated to try under desperate circumstances. Tense babies are made even more upset by tense arms, and they can read the tension in your face. What's good for mum is usually good for baby. Relaxation is contagious. If baby senses you're relaxed, she's likely to catch the feeling.

difficult. Try winding up your mechanical sub in order to wind down a fussy baby. The tick-tocking sound plus the monotonous motion will sometimes settle an upset baby. Some newer swings even oscillate in a circular motion besides the traditional back-and-forth motion. It's best to borrow a swing or try one out on your baby at the shop to avoid investing in something that your baby will shun. While some high-need babies won't settle for less than the highest-tech swing (those that move in two planes, play lullabies, and have a plush seat), others will calm with a simpler swing that hangs from a door or porch frame. Some babies prefer these swings on ropes to the mechanical ones with their rigid supports; they like to sway in a circular motion besides swinging from front to back. Some babies don't like any type of swing; perhaps they get dizzy. In that case, it's back to the human swing.

We warn parents against overusing mechanical swings. A high-need baby, if he doesn't reject the device outright, will tend to bond strongly to a swing if he's put in it routinely. It's especially important for the high-need baby to bond to people, not things.

My baby liked the trio of singing, slinging, and swinging. I would wear her facing out in the sling while swinging on a playground swing and singing to her.

Research has shown that movement stimulates the growth of brain cells and contributes to the overall organization of a child's nervous system. Since, we believe, some high-need children act the way they do because of a disorganized nervous system, movement will help to organize their behaviour.

4. Motorway Fathering (or Mothering)

If you've tried several of the home-based tricks to settle baby and none have worked, take a ride. Place baby in a car seat and drive for at least twenty minutes, non-stop if you can. Then return home and carry the whole package (sleeping baby in the car seat) into your home.

I used motorway fathering at times to give Martha a much needed baby break. Sometimes Martha and I would take a drive together for some couple communication time as our moving baby drifted off to sleep. During other baby nap times, I would bring a pillow along. After our baby fell asleep in the backseat, I would return to our driveway, park, and stretch out on the front seat for a bit of recharging before the household put more demands on me.

During one car ride my partner and I carried on an entire conversation to the tune of "Swing Low, Sweet Chariot" so that our baby would stay happy and we could get some important communicating done.

5. Strolling with a Pram

For many modern mothers, wearing babies in carriers has replaced pushing them in carriages. Certainly babies would give two thumbs up to this improved mode of travel. However, while most babies settle better when worn than when wheeled, some high-need babies like a change of scenery and sometimes settle better in a pram or buggy. Some infants shun the fixed-wheel, rough-riding buggies and prefer the old-fashioned, bouncy prams with springs. That's typical of high-need children.

One day we were doing a video shoot for the CD-ROM version of *The Baby Book*. From my paediatric practice, I had gathered a group of parents and their babies as models for this week-long project. (Bear in mind these were savvy parents and smart babies who had by this time worked out a style of parenting that met everyone's needs.) The producers wanted to show a couple out exercising together, with their baby in a jogging buggy. The selective little creature who had been cast for this scene refused to go into the buggy. She looked up at her mother, peered at the strange buggy, and gave the photographers a look of "I'm no dummy. Why should I settle for that contraption when I can travel first-class on mum?" The cameramen got the point. They realized they'd have to put a plastic baby in the buggy if they really wanted that shot. Plastic in plastic. That made more sense.

■ **WARNING:** prams are designed to soothe babies and sometimes get them to sleep, but it is not safe to leave baby sleeping in a pram unattended unless he is on his back or side and there are no pillows, extra blankets, or large plush toys to occlude baby's breathing. Some infants have smothered while left sleeping unattended in a pram.

6. Rolling Baby

Kneel on the floor and drape baby tummy-down over a beach ball. Hold baby with one hand and slightly roll the ball from side to side.

7. Bouncing Baby

Put baby on his stomach over your knees while you're sitting and bounce or jiggle your knees while patting baby's back. If you are lying down you can get the same effect by putting baby over your stomach and bouncing your bottom on the bed while patting.

Another way to bounce baby (and get eye contact going) is to hold baby in your hands with your arms away from your body. Use one hand under baby's bottom and the other hand and forearm supporting baby's neck and back. Then use an up-and-down bouncing motion with

happy hour!

Many fussy or colicky babies seem to go to pieces in the late afternoon or early evening, just when your parental reserves are already drained. If your baby is a "P.M. fusser" around the same time each day, plan "happy hour" before baby's colic hour occurs. Treat baby and yourself to a late afternoon nap. Upon awakening, go into a relaxing ritual, such as a twenty-minute baby massage, followed by a forty-minute walk carrying baby in a sling. With this before-colic ritual, baby is conditioned at the same time each day to expect an hour of comfort rather than an hour of pain.

a checklist of 36 time-tested baby-calmers

- Wearing baby in a sling
- Ceiling fan; bathroom extractor fan
- Dancing with baby
- Sounds of vacuum cleaner, dishwasher, washing machine, tumble drier
- Swinging baby
- Car rides
- Showing baby your "silly face"
- Pushing baby in pram
- Magic mirror
- Taking a walk
- Fire in fireplace
- Bouncing on trampoline
- Gazing at traffic
- Breast-feeding while walking with baby
- Watching parent on exercise machine
- Draping baby over a beach ball
- Watching television or video
- Comfort sucking: nursing, dummies, sucking on the move
- Infant massage
- Warm fuzzy

- Music, tapes of womb sounds, heartbeats
- Neck nestle
- Echoing baby's cry
- Nestle nursing
- Tape recordings of baby's own cries
- A warm bath together
- Tick-tock of clock or pendulum swing of grandfather clock
- Colic carries
- Eliminating bothersome foods from mother's diet if breast-feeding, or changing formula (see Chapter 10)
- Singing lullabies
- Vibrating, humming gadgets wrapped in nappy or blanket
- Slowing down mother's lifestyle and changing her expectations
- Running water
- Tape of environmental sounds
- Creating the most peaceful home environment possible
- Metronome

your arms, varying the rhythm until you find the tempo baby likes. You can also do this while walking or dancing.

8. Walking with Baby

One of the easiest baby- and parent-calmers is a simple walk. When our babies were fussy and obviously needed a change of scenery, we borrowed a well-known motto: "When the going gets tough, the tough get going." Martha or I would nestle our baby in a sling and take a long walk, each time trying to vary the route and the attractions. We would walk past moving cars, moving people, trees, parks, children playing, up and down hills, along curvy paths, and often along the beach. Sometimes we began the day with a baby walk, which seemed to start the day off better for both of us. Other times, when our babies were going through the stage when they fussed a lot around dinnertime, we would take a walk around five o'clock, which sometimes mellowed them out enough that they would reward us by forgetting to fuss that evening. Besides calming fussy babies, long, brisk walks are relaxing for parents since exercise releases endorphins, the body's natural relaxing hormones.

We have always believed that if our babies were going to fuss, they may as well fuss outside. Feeling housebound with a fussy baby is a double punishment that few parents can tolerate. This is especially true for those persistent P.M. fussers who need a half hour to an hour each evening to blow off steam. In that case, they may as well have their evening blast amid a change of scenery for you.

Taking a walk is good therapy for a mother who is struggling with burnout. A mother who is having trouble managing her new life and who also has a high-need baby is at risk for serious postpartum depression or high levels of anxiety. This mother-baby pair needs to be out of the house, walking briskly for at least an hour in the morning and again later in the day. Mother may worry that she's away from the house, "not getting enough done". "Home" to a baby is where mother is, and what she is doing is important. Walking will calm both mother and baby, and the exercise releases substances in the brain that soothe emotional and mental distress. Walking can help a new mother settle into a balanced and peaceful life so that she can reflect balance and peace to her baby.

9. Colic Carries

Here are some time-tested holds for putting a tense baby in relaxed arms:

Arm drapes. Rest baby's head in the crook of your elbow; drape baby's stomach along your forearm and grasp the nappy area firmly. Your forearm will press against baby's tense abdomen. When baby's tense limbs dangle instead of stretch out, baby is beginning to relax.

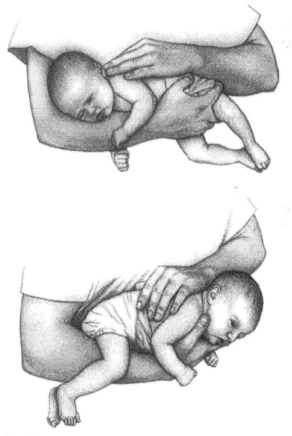

Arm drape.

For variety, try reversing this position, with baby's cheek in the palm of your hand and her nappy area in the crook of your elbow.

Colic curls. Babies who tense their tummy and arch their back often settle in this position. Slide baby's back down your chest and encircle your arms under his bottom. Curl baby up, facing forward with his head and back resting against your chest. As an added gas reliever, try

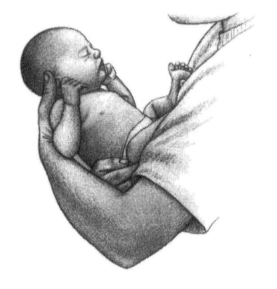

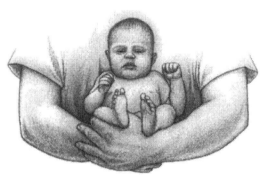

Colic curl.

pumping baby's thighs in a bicycle motion. Or try reversing the forward-facing position: baby's feet up against your chest as you hold him. In this position, you can maintain eye contact with your baby.

The handstand (beginning around age four months). Let baby face forward with his back up against your chest as he stands on one of your hands. Lean slightly back to discourage baby from lunging forward and keep the other hand planted firmly on baby's tummy to hold him securely and to add warmth and pressure to help his abdomen relax. The combination of the visual attractions of facing forward plus the concentration needed for baby to remain standing often causes baby to forget to fuss. The handstand also works well with baby resting against you chest-to-chest, his head peering

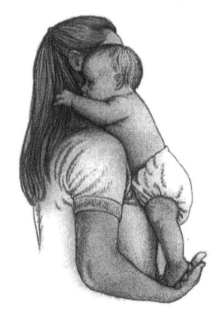

Handstand.

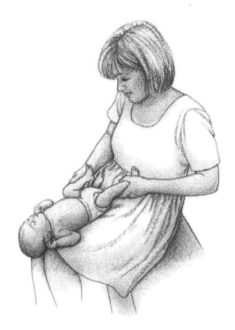

Lap pump.

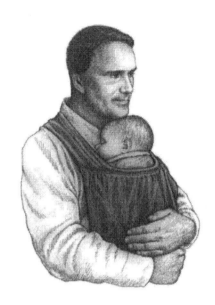

over your shoulder; there's also less chance of baby lunging forward out of your arms this way.

The lap pump. Lay baby on her back on your lap with her legs toward you and her head resting on your knees. Pump her legs up and down in a bicycling motion, while adding a few attention-getting facial antics.

The neck nestle. See page 74.

For added comforting and sleep-inducing success, try these holds while walking or dancing with your baby. Add soothing sounds and moving attractions, such as beaches, water running in the kitchen sink, or moving traffic.

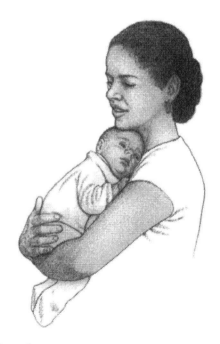

Neck nestle.

sounds that soothe

Along with motion, most babies are soothed by sounds, preferably ones that remind them of the womb. The most calming sounds are rhythmic, monotonous, low-pitched, and humming in quality, with slowly rising crescendos and decrescendos, and a sound pattern that repeats at a rate of sixty to seventy beats per minute. Infant-product manufacturers have capitalized on research into soothing sounds by producing a variety of sleep-inducing sound makers that use "white noise" – a monotonous, repetitive sound involving all the frequencies audible to the human ear; this will lull an overloaded mind into sleep. However, you don't need to go out and buy a special tape or gadget to lull your baby to sleep. Here are some proven baby-calming favourites that you may have around the house:

1. a loudly ticking clock
2. running or dripping water from a tap or shower
3. a vacuum cleaner (wear baby in a sling while vacuuming). If baby likes the sound of the vacuum cleaner, you can save wear and tear on the machine by making a tape recording of the sound and playing the tape instead of running the vacuum. Some infants, however, panic at vacuum cleaner-like sounds.
4. a bathroom extractor fan with light turned out
5. a fan or dishwasher
6. a metronome set at sixty beats per minute
7. a tape recording of a waterfall or ocean waves or running tap
8. homemade lullabies. Babies settle best with slowly rising and falling melodies with repetitive themes that gradually fade away. Pick a simple tune (for example, "Frère Jacques") and make up simple words:

> *Time for sleeping, time for sleeping,*
> *Jason dear, Jason dear.*
> *Mummy's very tired, Mummy's very tired,*
> *Go to sleep, go to sleep.*

You can put Daddy in for Mummy's name in the next verse, or change another line in a small way. These variations can go on for a long time, and it takes no musical skill at all to create this kind of personal theme song for your baby. Tape recordings of your own voice are especially helpful to soothe your baby when she is left in the care of a sub.

9. a homemade medley. Pick out songs on various tapes that baby likes (and that you like), and using a duplicating tape recorder, make one tape containing a medley of favourite soothing tunes.
10. "settle-best" music. Most babies like classical music with steady tempos and slowly rising and falling dynamics, such as Mozart and Vivaldi. Many relax to quieter music, such as classical guitar and flute. A musical box playing Brahms's Lullaby is a time-honoured baby settler. Sometimes playing easy-listening music all day long helped our older babies have more relaxed days (us, too!). A CD player on repeat is especially helpful to replay a favourite medley of lullabies for an impatient baby who goes to pieces if he must wait for a parent to change the CD. Be sure to

choose music that you like listening to, because you're going to hear it over and over. In general, rock music or any music that does not have an easily perceived melody is too turbulent for babies and often aggravates an already tense baby. Other music that may be soothing to your baby includes the music you relaxed to during pregnancy and massage music available from your local massage instructor.

11. a tape recording of your baby's own cry. Played at the onset of a fuss, your baby's own cry can take him by surprise, quieting him long enough for you to get through to him with another distraction. One mother would echo the crying sound directly back to her baby when he began to cry uncontrollably.

12. the hum and slosh of a washing machine. One desperate mother secured her baby in a car seat on top of an automatic washer while it was running. Baby always drifted off to sleep. You should take the car seat off the machine once baby is asleep. NEVER LEAVE BABY UNATTENDED IN THIS PRECARIOUS SITUATION. The car seat can easily vibrate right off the machine.

I don't like to hear rock music at full blast around babies. I know a mother who let her husband do this and she has three of the most violent children I know.

Sounds to avoid. As a baby, Hayden trained us never to turn on the blender or the mixer when she was in the room. If we had to use these tools, we had to first make sure she could be occupied elsewhere in the house.

She hated the loud, sudden, high-pitched squeal of the motor, and responded with the sound of her own turned-on motor.

sights that delight

A captivating image can distract some babies in the midst of a crying fit and sidetrack others before they have a chance to howl. Try these:

1. Magic Mirror

This scene has pulled our babies out of many crying jags. Hold the fussy baby in front of a mirror and let her witness her own drama. Place her hand or bare foot against its image on the mirror surface and watch the intrigued baby grow silent.

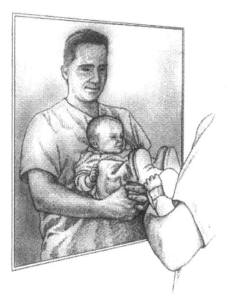

Magic mirror.

no problem!

One of the "joys" of sailing is that something usually goes wrong, requiring outside help. A recent sailing vacation in the Caribbean found us once again limping into port with our chartered boat, asking knowledgeable natives for assistance. Our anxiety was immediately relieved by the usual Caribbean response, "No problem, mon!" This attitude relaxed us. If there was no problem, then there was no need to worry. We have dubbed this relaxed approach to problem solving "the Caribbean attitude". This Caribbean attitude also works on fussy babies.

Kristy brought her ten-month-old baby, Maisie, to my surgery for high-need-baby counselling. As soon as Kristy put Maisie down on the floor, Maisie would fuss to be picked up. Within a millisecond of her first peep, Kristy lunged for Maisie and scooped her up into her arms. Baby's anxiety triggered mother's anxiety, which then reinforced baby's fussiness, and they became one anxious pair.

I explained to Kristy that she was giving Maisie the message that there really was a reason to fuss. Instead, I suggested she try conveying the "no problem" message. She should continue to converse with me, wearing her relaxed face. When Maisie started to fuss, she should turn toward her and briefly acknowledge her, still with a relaxed, happy face, and then resume the conversation as if no problem existed. Kristy tried this and was amazed that Maisie stopped fussing and began crawling around the room playing on her own. Mother had conveyed to her, "no problem, baby; no need to fuss".

2. Happy Face

Spend a lot of time in face-to-face contact with your baby, showing baby exaggerated (but pleasant) facial expressions. Remember which facial expressions he likes and replay them later when he fusses. High-need babies demand a lot of connecting experiences, and face-to-face, eye-to-eye contact is what they need in order to know they are being heard and seen clearly. Give baby a sudden change of face. Put on your silliest or most dramatic facial gestures and direct them at baby. These antics take baby by

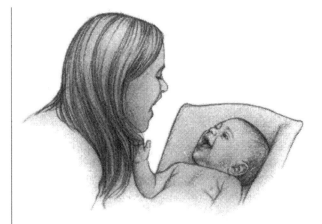

Happy face.

surprise, causing him (at least temporarily) to forget why he is fussing. All this connecting is why high-need babies grow up to be such good communicators, sensitive to the body language and nonverbal cues of others. They get plenty of practice.

Also, know when to back off. Constant or sudden intense in-your-face confrontations can make babies anxious.

3. Miscellaneous Moving Attractions

Seldom do you have to buy stuff to hush little babies. You'll be amazed what natural babycalmers are all around your home. We've enjoyed placing our babies in front of these natural "visual stimulators":

- ceiling lights or chandeliers
- the swinging pendulum of a grandfather clock
- a shower (put baby in an infant seat and let him watch you in the shower)
- revolving ceiling fan
- aquarium
- running water
- leaves on trees (hold baby at the window or on the grass so she can gaze at the leaves swaying in the wind and their moving shadows on the grass)
- moving cars (place baby at the window so that he can see the cars zooming past)
- waves on the beach
- metronome
- children playing
- pets playing
- fire in fireplaces

The more interactions you try, the better you become at comforting your baby, and you'll have some fun along the way. One father tried everything until he discovered his baby would stop fussing when watching a popcorn popper in action.

touches that relax

1. Infant Massage

High-need babies have tense muscles that need help relaxing. Every baby needs lots of touching. High-need babies need more (of course!). There is no touch more soothing than that of skin on skin, although for some babies, skin-to-skin contact can actually be experienced as stimulating, so you have to proceed with caution. Infants who spend time in neonatal intensive care units after birth tend to have a high need for pleasant touch, since so much of the touching they experienced in the hospital was painful. Some very sensitive high-need babies actually pull away from being touched because they find it threatening or over-stimulating. In this case, a routine of careful, gentle touches can gradually accustom this baby to being handled and will help him eventually enjoy touching.

Infant massage is an enjoyable way to touch and soothe your infant. You can learn the art of infant massage from an infant massage instructor. (Ask your health visitor, midwife or NCT antenatal teacher to recommend someone.) An instructor can be especially helpful if your baby seems to be over-stimulated by touching. You can also teach yourself, using the instruction manual *Infant Massage: A Handbook for Loving Parents*, by Vimala McClure (Souvenir Press, 2001). For more information on infant massage, try http://www.iaim.org.uk.

2. The Warm Fuzzy

Here's a high-touch soother where father can really shine. Dads, lie down and drape baby skin-to-skin over your chest, placing baby's ear over your heart. As baby senses the rhythm of your heartbeat plus the up-and-down motion of your breathing, you will feel the tense baby relax. His fists will uncurl and his limbs will dangle limply over your chest. By the time baby is three or four months of age, he may squirm and easily roll off your chest. Try letting your baby nestle against you with the top of his head in your armpit, his tummy resting comfortably against the side of your chest. In this position, baby's ear can still hear your heartbeat and sense your steady breathing. Pat his nappy gently with your free hand to reinforce the calm feeling.

3. The Neck Nestle

Here is another high-touch baby-calmer where dad shines. While walking, dancing, or lying with your baby on your chest, snuggle her head against the front of your neck and drape your chin over baby's head. Then hum or sing a low-pitched melody like "Old Man River" while swaying from side to side. The vibration of your voice box and jaw against your baby's sensitive skull can often lull the tense baby right to sleep.

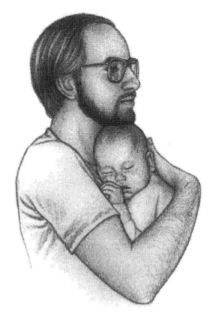

Neck nestle.

Some of my most memorable moments as the father of infants are of holding my babies in the neck nestle position while singing the Sears family's "Go to Sleep" song to the tune of Brahms's Lullaby:

> *Go to sleep, go to sleep,*
> *Go to sleep my little baby.*
> *Go to sleep, go to sleep,*
> *Go to sleep my little girl.*

4. Nestle Nursing

Undress your baby down to a nappy and lie down on the bed together. Curl up womblike around your baby, face-to-face, tummy-to-tummy, or let the baby feed. This is especially nice if mum's clothing allows for lots of skin contact. The natural calming powers of touching, sucking, your breathing and heartbeat, along with gentle strokes from your fingers, will relax even the fussiest baby and send her off into peaceful sleep. Martha calls this hold the "teddy bear snuggle".

5. A Warm Bath Together

This one's for mother and baby. Mothers of high-need babies have put in a lot of hours of hydrotherapy because it works! Recline in a half-full bath, and have dad hand baby to you. If you are alone, have baby "stand by" in an infant seat right next to the bath until you are ready to bring her into the bath. Place baby tummy-to-tummy against your chest and let baby breast-feed in the water (your nipples being a couple of inches above the surface). Baby is floating a bit while feeding, which adds to the soothing effect. Taking a bath with baby helps to relax mum as well as baby. Leave the tap running and the bath's drain open a bit. The drip of the warm water not only provides a soothing sound, but also keeps the water comfortably warm.

Getting the sleeping baby out of the bath is a bit of a challenge. Some babies will stay asleep while they are handed to someone waiting with a warm, dry towel. Most high-need babies don't sleep through handovers, however. You just may have to plan to stay in the bath for a while. Have some relaxing music on that you can enjoy. Or have a book handy (this may or may not work, depending on the design of your bath). If you really don't want to stay in the bath the whole time baby sleeps, and he doesn't pass well to someone (or if you're alone), plan your strategy for getting both of you out of the bath and resettled on your bed. Have the infant seat next to the bath with the warm, dry towel draped over it. (Try having a hot water bottle there keeping the towel warm until you're ready to place baby on the towel.) If baby wakes up during this transfer, don't despair. Wrap yourself up in your own big, fluffy bath sheet, pick baby up calmly, and head for your bed. Snuggle up together with as little fuss as possible, and baby may obligingly feed back off to sleep for you.

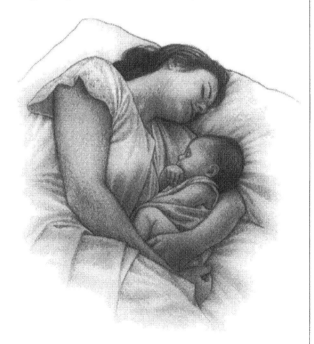

Teddy bear snuggle.

free-choice sucking

If baby strongly resists or refuses sucking, don't force it on her. The goal here is to help baby, not overpower her. She may need to let off steam for a while before she can accept the nipple. By forcing the nipple into her mouth, you would be teaching her that she has absolutely no power or right to express her feelings. You would be forcing her to ignore her need to just wail for a while. Comfort her just enough to help her, so that she can make the choice to stop crying. That is healthy. Do not allow yourself to become so overburdened with baby and the rest of your life that you resort to forced comforting in an attempt to get some peace and quiet. If lack of sleep is doing this to you, find help with older children or ease up on household projects so that you can nap whenever baby sleeps. If your own inner panic about baby's crying is making you feel this way, get some professional help in understanding and dealing with this panic.

It's pretty hard to force a baby to suck on your breast, because a baby must actively latch on in order to feed. But you can force a rigid, rubber nipple into a reluctant baby's mouth. Once a tiny baby feels the nipple on his palate, he has to suck – it's a reflex. A determined mother can force a newborn to suck just by shoving the dummy into place. This is one reason we don't like dummies. (Actually, even a breast-feeding mother could do this if she tried hard enough.)

It's important for a mother to discern whether the baby wants to suck or wants to cry. A little teasing and enticement to take the nipple is okay as long as you are calm and relaxed. Even a little cajoling won't cross over the line into the forcing category as long as your goal is really to help the baby, not to shut him up because you can't handle the crying. If your nipples are wearing out, you can encourage baby to suck on your finger. While sucking is an easy answer to infant crying, don't let it be the only tool in your bag of comforting tricks. Study all the possibilities and be open to what your baby is telling you.

chapter 5

feelings shared by parents of high-need children

The child you got may not be the child you expected. Along with parenting a high-need child come feelings you never expected to have. Doubt, worry, and frustration are common among parents of high-need babies. By understanding why you have these feelings, you can better manage yourself so that you can better manage your child.

Learning to manage these feelings can be a growth process for you, one that carries over into other areas of your life.

doubtful

Having a high-need baby sets you up to question your parenting abilities. You watch other parents and their babies. Their babies sleep through the night; yours awakens frequently. Their babies lie quietly in the cot; yours will settle for nothing less than your arms. You begin to wonder if other parents are doing something right and you're doing something wrong.

Then comes the parade of baby-care advisers sharing their personal "you shoulds", all of which give you the not-so-subtle message that your baby acts this way because of something you are doing wrong. In a result-oriented society, even the most independent woman begins to doubt her mothering when her baby does not act like the neighbourhood norm. Whatever confidence you have left is further shaken when nothing you do seems to be working.

Though we were dedicated to being attached parents, there were times when we felt discouraged and alone in our beliefs. Everywhere we looked, experts, authors, paediatricians, and other parents were telling us how to "condition" our baby to sleep through the night and to self-soothe. We would look at other new parents and remark on how calm their babies seemed. In the height of his colic, we would find ourselves secretly wishing that Tom could be that way.

Though we knew he was his own unique self, we were in a very confusing predicament, pitting what we instinctively believed to be right against what we saw was apparently working for other people. We could have taken the easier, more popular route. We could have bought a cot and let him cry, and we would have received all kinds of immediate reinforcement from those around us. But we knew if we did that, we would not only be abandoning our fundamental beliefs but also making choices based on our own needs, not Tom's. It was important to hold his interests above our temporary need for reinforcement and security. After all, it was his life we needed to respect with the choices we made.

As new parents struggling to forge a different way, we were going on pure faith and gut feelings most of the time, trying everything that felt right but never knowing for certain if it was helping or working. In the beginning, there were no "results" to let us know that we were on the right track – not even so much as a sign pointing out the general direction in which we were supposed to go. Because we were seeing immediate results for other people's kids, we questioned whether our method would even work in the long run. While what we saw and heard from many of the experts "guaranteed" certain (short-term) results, our approach required faith and trust in long-term benefits. There were times when, out of sheer desperation, we would try an alternative approach and hesitantly employ the techniques that the method prescribed. Without fail, it was promptly discarded because it conflicted with our basic beliefs about parenting and never really addressed Tom's needs specifically. It was (and

still is) important for us to give Tom what he was "telling" us he needed. Employing some technique that tried to change him in some fundamental way seemed counterproductive and just plain wrong.

Believing in attachment parenting wasn't always easy. When times were especially rough, we'd read and reread various chapters in The Baby Book, *which helped to reinforce our commitment. Then, inevitably, we would hear some "expert" on television describe a quick and easy way to "solve" our problem and we would feel completely lost again. We now realize that all of our going back and forth, questioning and re-evaluating, helped us to forge an even stronger confidence in our own knowing.*

In many ways, attachment parenting has not been the easy way to go. It requires faith and trust and a certain strength of conviction to remain firm in light of all the other popular messages. But, in every way, it has been the most life-affirming, soulful way to go. Taking the road less travelled has made all the difference.

alone

Even when you find a parenting style that works, you may feel alone in your circle of friends. Because your child has different needs, your parenting will naturally be different. You may find yourself increasingly reluctant to ask for an understanding ear, fearing you will get judgment or unwanted advice instead. Because your child may be especially needy during social gatherings, you find yourself always making excuses for her behaviour, and you become increasingly resentful of "those looks" from less sympathetic friends. As you sit in the Mother and Toddler groups, searching for adult companionship, you feel like retreating to the bathroom, as yours seems to be the only baby who constantly demands attention. Eventually, you make excuses and avoid these groups, convinced that you don't belong among these perfect mothers with perfect children. You could become a recluse, resigned to your plight, and resenting it.

Some days I feel so lost. Perhaps it's the tremendous exhaustion and lack of sleep or personal space. Perhaps it's that she seems to need physical and emotional contact the most when I've slept the least. I feel so alone in this. There is no feminine lexicon to guide me. Extended family is scattered … no support, no advice. I am left solely to my own devices with this child who knows more about what's going on than I do. I want to scream sometimes. I want to run so desperately. I defend myself stalwartly against inadequacy. I fantasize about a different life and feel bad about all of it. I seem to have no internal standards of rightness: how do I feel about it all? All I know is that my life is so very different now and I have no place to hide from the frustration and pain and rage. I just wish I could be sure I was doing the right thing.

defensive

One of the most gnawing aggravations that go along with high-need parenting is fending off unhelpful advice from pestering friends. You will feel embarrassed when yours is the only baby who won't settle for the sitters in the church crèche, and angry when advisers admonish you for always "giving in" to your baby.

Attachment parenting is, for most of us, a lonely, bumpy road. When talking to paediatricians and other parents, we don't know how much we can reveal because we don't know whether they share the same philosophical beliefs about parenting. For the first six months of Helen's life, we went on blind faith alone: faith in our deepest sense that this was the right way to go. Now she is ten months old and we are seeing the benefits of attachment parenting in full bloom. Folks who know her say she is "serene" and yet so full of animation and life. She is full of a kind of joy that seems rooted in a deep sense of security. Attachment parenting has given us the structure and validation we needed to become exactly the kind of parents we wanted to be. I would not say that this is the easiest way to go. It requires a lot of energy and openness and vulnerability. The process of attachment parenting has caused us to open ourselves to Helen, to the unknown, and to who she needs to be. Being that available to another person opens up spaces in yourself that have been unknowingly locked away. Both my husband and I have noticed changes in ourselves on the deepest levels that we can only attribute to parenting a high-need child. Parenting is truly a spiritual and psychological journey.

As a result of all of this, we now find that popular messages about parenting today make us profoundly sad. At what point in this country did we start putting such an outrageous premium on independence? We seem to want small babies to be "easy" and extremely self-sufficient. Is it because no one has time to parent anymore, or is it because we've forgotten that it's okay (even necessary) to need other people? We see articles and talk show segments every day promoting "training" six-week-old breast-fed babies to sleep through the night; new gadgets that simulate human contact; day care; early weaning – it goes on and on. Is it any wonder that we are becoming a society of angry, addicted, and lonely people? It seems to us that the key to solving many of the big, complicated social problems is for parents to

be able to devote themselves to the parenting of their children, to raising children who are so full of rightness and self-esteem that as adults they have no need for unhealthy behaviours to fill up the spaces where love should have been.

for better or for worse ...

The experience of parenting a high-need child can be an asset or a liability. Depending on your attitude, living with a high-need child can become an opportunity for growth, a chance to hone your skills, sharpen your sensitivity, and even smooth some rough edges in your own personality. One of the statements we hear most frequently from parents of high-need children is, "This experience has made me a better parent, and a better person." Or, it can be a negative experience, full of conflict and wishing that your child was anything but the person she really is. Your child's personality is not in your control, but whether your experience is generally positive or negative is up to you.

resentful

Why me? Why my baby? "Other babies eat and sleep. Mine eats all the time and never sleeps." You resent your plight. What's worse, you resent yourself for having such unmotherly feelings. It's hard to keep the new-parent glow when you're sleep-deprived. It's hard to "think positive" when every time you sit down to a long-awaited, romantic dinner with your partner-turned-stranger, your baby wails just as you're lighting the candles.

It helped when we finally understood that we didn't get a "bad" baby (and that we weren't "bad" parents). Now we are more confident about sticking to our convictions and intuitions. Other people have only to be with Karen to know that we are doing what is right for her and right for us.

● ● ●

I expected to have a darling baby who would just eat and sleep for those early weeks. How misguided I was. Mine just ate.

thrilled and scared

While living with a high-need baby, there will be high moments when your child's unique personality shines and you count your blessings to be the parent of such a special person. Other times you'll plunge into despair and would gladly swap for that easy baby next door. The uneven temperament of these babies keeps you always guessing. You are constantly challenged physically and emotionally. Early mornings may be particularly stressful; upon awakening, you don't know whether this is going to be a great day or a dreadful one. The great days you wouldn't trade for a million pounds. Many parents describe life with a high-need baby as riding a roller coaster.

At the end of the movie *Parenthood*, the grandmother tells a story about how, as a young girl, she loved riding the roller coaster: "Up, down. Up, down. Oh, what a ride! I always wanted to go again. You know, it was just interesting to me that a ride could make me so frightened, so scared, so sick, so, so excited, and so thrilled – all together. Some didn't like it. They went on the merry-go-round. That just goes around – nothing. I liked the roller coaster. You get more out of it."

controlled

Most of us enter parenthood expecting to be in control of our baby, or at least in charge. You expect the baby to respond to you, to follow your lead. You call the shots. You set the daily routine. You determine where baby sleeps and when baby is in your arms or in his cot. Now you find yourself losing control – of yourself and your baby. You discover it's a myth that good parents are always in control – or you wonder if perhaps you are not good parents.

Not only do you feel that you're not controlling your infant, what's worse, you imagine he's controlling you. And at every gathering, there is always a band of well-meaning advisers reinforcing this fear. You plan your day to suit your mood, only to find out you need to change plans to fit your child's mood. It's inconvenient for you to shop in the morning, but you know that taking your two-year-old shopping at four in the afternoon (on the way home from all the other errands) invites disaster. You're in a playgroup and it's time to go. While other toddlers willingly comply with their mothers' departure announcements, your child protests and dissolves into a tantrum. Your authority is on the line. You look around imagining that all your friends are shaking their heads, wondering why you can't control your child. Another blow to your maternal honour.

I never felt in control. I'd feel like everything was going okay and then something would set Wendy off, and we'd begin a downhill slide. If I had plans for the day, I'd have to abandon them because I knew that we would have a miserable time. I'm a type A personality, and I think that it is a lot harder on mothers like me who have high expectations, low flexibility, and a general need to be in control. I would also feel isolated as a result of not being able to go out with my baby like all my friends, and embarrassed when I'd have to explain why I was cancelling an outing. That isolation then added another burden to my already mentally and physically exhausted body. (What I've since learned is that Wendy is also a type A personality, and our personalities often clash, which means we must work hard to manage our relationship.) I also felt I was being manipulated. Although this is a control-related issue, it's important that now, ten years later, I can safely say that I was not being manipulated as much as I thought. I had a high-need baby who had needs beyond the normal scope that had to be met in order for her to feel safe and secure. At the time, though, it brought on much anguish.

critical

As you work through the feelings of "Why me?" "Why my baby?", you might start blaming people and circumstances for your plight. Looking for targets to blame is a natural part of searching for answers, yet this process usually adds more questions than it answers. You seldom find a source to pin the problem on. Here's how one mother worked through her blame:

I blamed myself. I blamed the hospital. I blamed her prematurity. Then I got into a whole litany of "if onlys, if onlys". If only I had carried her to term, been able to hold her more, et cetera. I felt that I could have changed conditions to make it better for her. Those feelings are still there, but I realize the futility in dwelling on them. I finally came to the realization that Meghan is a fussy baby, and I

needed to find ways to cope with her fussiness and relieve it as much as possible. I often felt angry with myself and frustrated with her. I had angry feelings I never had had before. For the first time in my life I could understand child abuse, and believe me, that scared me. I would be so angry with her for crying and crying that I would then yell at my three-year-old for something really minor. When my husband got home, boy! did he get it if he stepped out of line. I never abused my baby, but I was mean to our three-year-old and my husband by yelling at them. After getting some counselling, I realized I couldn't do everything perfectly all the time for everyone, and had to stop trying. I wasn't supermum and I wasn't born on the planet Krypton. My counsellor advised me to leave Meghan for an hour or so every week and do something for myself, but she knew that I wouldn't follow this advice. I compromised by hiring a teen to come in and play with Meghan and Katie for two hours, two times a week, while I was in another room reading or doing whatever I chose to do. That way if Meghan needed me, I'd be there.

Eventually you will come to the conclusion that there is no one at whom to aim the blame. You have a high-need baby through no one's fault, least of all yours. Here is how one mother put this realization into words:

I had an uncomplicated, healthy pregnancy, during which I took meticulous care of myself, read all the right books, and did everything as naturally as possible. I had an unmedicated, satisfying birth, went home after three hours, immediately bonding. I got every item on my wish list. Even our home is calm. We have no smoking, no TV. We are calm parents, and even the dog is gentle. We play lots of classical music. We live in clean air on eight acres of forest. He is still a high-need baby.

tied down

Often new mothers, especially when moving from career to full-time baby care, tell us they feel so tied down. Yes, you will feel tied down. It is a new way of life for you, and this is a very natural reaction. High-need babies don't readily accept substitute caregivers. The incessant demands of your baby necessitate getting out beyond your four walls for some space and adult companionship. Yet the same neediness of your baby makes it difficult for you to go out in public. Sometimes you feel trapped into meeting your baby's needs because that's what's expected of you as a mother. Perhaps during your pregnancy you made a decision to put your career on the back burner temporarily and devote yourself to a new full-time career as a mother. You wanted to give yourself entirely to your baby and meet her needs; now you're afraid you may go crazy at home unless some of your grown-up needs are met.

I was jealous of other mothers whose babies could be left, could sit and play or look at books and enjoy doing so. I felt so tied down because I could do nothing without her and because no one else could care for her. I would get angry at her for

being so difficult, and angry and confused at myself for getting angry, and also angry wondering if I had raised her to be this way. By the end of the day I was drained from frustration and guilt and would dump her on my husband when he walked in the door. When I woke up in the morning I would suddenly feel a great burden of frustration of "here we go again".

The more tired I was, the more frustrated and tearful I became. Sometimes I felt trapped and resentful, especially when I compared Katie to my friends' babies, who were much more easygoing. I imagined that I would never again be able to do anything except hold my baby. I felt like throwing her away or running away myself. Yet I was so in love with Katie I could hardly believe I would have such thoughts. They made me feel guilty, and I wondered if I was a bad mother.

● ● ●

I gradually went from feeling tied down to tied together. It helped when I realized this high-need stage was a short time in our lives. I can always play tennis later.

inadequate

Baby cries, mother comforts, baby quiets. Baby feels loved, mother feels capable, both feel good. That's the scene you envision. Yet there are days when nothing seems to comfort your baby. And then, just when you've reached the end of your baby-soothing rope, your infant has a happy day – only you don't know why. Was it the early nap?

Was it the late-afternoon car trip? The visit from Grandma? Two days later, the calm is broken by a storm and baby is back to his old behaviour again, affirming what you suspected all along – something is wrong with your baby, and something is wrong with your mothering.

Going places with Eileen seemed like all work and no fun. She didn't enjoy leaving the house (although the car ride in the car seat did offer some pleasure if we were moving and not caught in a traffic jam). After arriving, the unfamiliar surroundings would seem more than she could handle. Too much stimulation of any kind upset her system, and the hysteria would set in. When brave enough to attempt a restaurant, we tried to pick loud family ones so that her expected crying and discontent could be drowned out by the jukebox and chatter. Many times it wasn't worth the effort because I would be met by disapproving stares from mothers who obviously knew how to quiet their babies. Church was a joke. The nursery didn't want her, and we certainly couldn't sit "quietly" in the back row. Again, feelings of guilt and inadequacy.

• • •

No matter how hard I tried, I kept feeling (reinforced by other people) it was my fault that my baby fussed. In my before-mother-hood career, I had always been able to set goals and achieve them. This time I could not make my baby happy.

lost

You keep giving, baby keeps taking, and you feel like giving out. Fatigue compounds all the other feelings of inadequacy, anger, and the realization that motherhood is not always the day-long joyful experience you had envisioned. The more tired you are, the less effective you become as a baby-comforter, and baby fusses more. Your fatigue affects your other roles. You become "touched-out" as a wife (less than thrilled when your mate wants physical intimacy – you've had all the touching you need from baby all day long), unable to concentrate at work, and your social life dwindles to fleeting encounters with a few fussy baby-tolerant friends. There will be times when you feel a complete loss of your sense of self.

For me, having a high-need baby was a test of endurance and stamina. Was there enough of me to go around? Could I still be as present and engaged as I wanted to be with so little sleep? It has taught me lessons about my own physical limitations. Having a child who requires a high level of parenting is demanding physically, mentally, and emotionally. There were times, especially during periods of her rapid growth, when I began to feel almost transparent ... like I didn't really exist. I spent so much of my time being present for the baby and for Steve that my own presence didn't receive much (if any) of my attention. As a result, I felt more and more depleted as each day passed until one day I suddenly burst into tears. It took a near breakdown for me to realize that I needed to pay

a lesson in self-awareness

Parenting a high-need child takes you on a journey of personal discovery into how you were parented. Also, it uncovers your strengths and weaknesses and forces you into a realistic appraisal of yourself. When your baby cries – for the third time that night – your first reaction betrays your real feelings. If your first thought is "another disruption, another inconvenience, another tired tomorrow …" it may be your own needy self rising up, wishing someone were taking care of you. Since none of us got perfectly responsive parenting (that's life!), we all will have this thought to some extent. But now that we are the parents, it's up to us somehow to be responsive. That is our job description. In order to do that, many of us must find a way to heal the areas of need within ourselves.

As you face this job and begin to be aware of and care for your own needs, you will find that you start to focus less on yourself and more on your baby: "How can I help her settle when she wakes up?" This is an appropriate focus when you are parenting a young infant. A high-need baby will keep your attention mostly on her for longer than most babies, but you will find that healthy responsiveness is the road to maturity for yourself as well as for your baby. Mothers have confided to us that they find parenting a high-need baby therapeutic: "it's the first time in my whole life I think of anyone else's needs first". Other mothers discover that caring for a needy baby helps them get in touch with deep needs of their own: "I've had to learn to manage my own inner self, and be sure to attend to my own needs for peace and balance, so that I could truly be the calm, mature mother my baby needs."

more attention to myself, and yet I really didn't know how to do that. I was so focused on being a mother that it seemed difficult (if not impossible) to change hats and focus on being an individual person.

It took me several more tearful breakdowns to realize what the problem really was and what I could do to change things. I looked at why I felt so drained of energy. I felt like it was being siphoned out of me until there was none left. I suspected that it was probable, given my perfectionist tendencies, that I was trying too hard to be

present and available for my family. I realized that when my focus was on them, I had no awareness of myself as a physical presence. There was only my awareness of them. All of my energy and focus was directed outward. I decided to begin being conscious of my breathing and the feeling of my feet on the floor while I watched Amy play or fed her lunch. I began to be consciously aware of myself, my own physical presence, while I was with others. It is not that I have reduced the amount of attention I give to Amy or Steve but that I acknowledge that I exist too in this relationship.

worried

When your baby acts differently from other babies, it's normal to wonder if something is wrong with her: "Could this be more than a passing stage?" "Could she have some painful illness?" Your mind wants a logical explanation for colicky or fussy behaviour, and you may go on searching for a physical cause despite reassurances from your doctor that your baby is healthy. (See Chapter 10, "Hidden Causes of Fussiness in Infants".)

I became a compulsive worrier. I questioned everything Maeve did as being a symptom or sign of a deep underlying problem. I was racked with feelings of depression and even went as far as to have her tested for HIV because she had had a blood transfusion at birth. I desperately needed an answer for this odd behaviour.

disillusioned

Many parents are not prepared for what life with a new baby is really like. Double that disillusionment when parenting a high-need baby. When Martha taught childbirth classes, she tried to paint a realistic picture of first-year parenting – the ups and downs, the days of unparalleled joy, and the days of sleepless fatigue. Yet she realized expectant couples hear only the positive parts of parenting, in the same way that they may visualize the ecstasy of the birth moment without thinking seriously about managing the labour to get there. They don't think realistically about what happens after they take baby home.

Mercifully, much of the first three months is a blur of walking, worrying, bouncing, singing, and crying. That was the most gruelling, heartbreaking thing we had ever gone through. It was not what we thought having a newborn child would be like. I had to throw out all the images of a mother quietly rocking her drowsy baby. Those babies on the formula commercials were not Lisa, and those mothers were not me.

• • •

When Amanda was born, I never dreamed that she would end up in my bed, that I would breast-feed her for more than two years, or that I wouldn't go out to the movies with my husband for over a year. My husband never expected to spend nights in another room, cook our breakfast every morning, or occasionally go to a movie alone. We had to learn to throw out our unrealistic expectations (such as husband and wife sleeping in the same bed every night while baby sleeps through the night in another room) and start from scratch, finding ways to meet everyone's needs.

manipulated

One of the most challenging parts of parenting the high-need child is deciding when to listen to the child's cues, trusting that the child knows best what she needs, and when to intervene to shape

s-t-r-e-t-c-h-e-d

During the early years of living with our first high-need child, I must have heard Martha use the term "stretched" a hundred times. Stretch is exactly what high-need children do to – and for – their parents. Yet, this powerful word has helpful and harmful meanings. Parenting a high-need child forces you to extend yourself, to re-evaluate priorities (sometimes even to change careers), to mature your mind-set about babies, and to become flexible and creative beyond your wildest dreams. Depending on your attitude toward raising a high-need child, the support you get, and the inner resources you have, repeated stretching can either wear you out, like a rubber band, or make you stronger, like a muscle. Yes, you do have to become flexible, almost elastic, in moment-by-moment high-need decisions, yet at what point do you have to guard against stretching until you snap?

Mothering is the most stressful job you will ever have. It's continual. The direction of the energy flow is constantly outward. Yet without challenges, no one grows in their profession, especially parents. The key is to get strong like a muscle, not weak like an overextended rubber band. Your life will never be the same. I remember tired parents in my surgery once saying, "We'll be happy when this high-need stage is over and our lives can get back to normal." I reminded them that as parents, from now on, this was their normal life. Becoming parents is like putting on a new pair of shoes. Through repeated wear you stretch them, and they gradually feel more comfortable; and the shoes, like life, are never again the same.

Sometimes I paint a rather grim picture of this high-need child. The reality is anything but grim. Certainly, I am very sleep-deprived and get exasperated when I get no breaks from the "action". However, Katherine is the most fascinating person I have ever met. She is extremely intelligent, and, while being demanding, seems to draw people to her. Her grandparents are completely captivated by her. Life is never boring with this little one. She is "on" almost all the time. She has taught me patience. I have learned many things because she challenges me to find new ways to deal with her demands. I have learned to enjoy the enormous amount of time I must spend with her. Interestingly, I don't like to be away from her more than a couple of hours. My friends can't understand why I don't want more breaks from her. Part of the reason I don't stay away from her for so long is I will have to "pay" for that time apart by her being more clingy and nursing more. But mostly I prefer to have her with me because I enjoy her company so much.

the child's behaviour, because in this particular situation you know best. This will be a play-by-play judgment, and expect it to be difficult. One of the main hurdles you will need to overcome is the issue of control. Many of us have entered our parenting career believing that good parents are always in control and that it is our job to take control of the child rather than let the child take the lead. The old fear of manipulation and spoiling will keep rearing its destructive head. It helps to think in terms of whose needs are greatest at a certain time and of being "responsive" rather than worrying about who is leading whom. This is the story of one set of parents who struggled with and solved this dilemma.

Deciding when to align ourselves with David and follow his lead and when to intervene has been a growth process for us. Intervention is sometimes a necessary step in helping him adapt to the world, but it can sometimes set up a relationship where he and we work against each other. My husband, Steve, experienced this during David's colic. There were times when Steve would try to bounce him down to sleep and David would struggle and strain; Steve would find himself fighting against David, trying to "break him down". This conflict-oriented approach never worked, nor did it feel right to Steve because he knew that he was trying to overpower David. Luckily, David, high-need child that he is, is a tough one to overpower. Over time, my husband learned that if he broke down his own resistance to the process and gave up the need to struggle, he was able to open himself up and work with David – with David's own needs and David's own rhythms – and he would invariably fall peacefully asleep.

Breaking down resistances came to be an important concept for us. We found that when we began fighting the way things were (for instance, when it was time for David to sleep and he wasn't going down), frustration, distance, and anger were certain to follow. If we instead allowed things to be just the way they were – no more, no less – things just flowed more easily. There was a feeling of peace and rightness. A wise Eastern philosophy warns against "pushing the river", and we found that it's much easier with a high-need baby to ignore the way we think things should be and simply "go with the flow".

We discovered this same outlook with our high-need babies, too, and having gone through the process of lowering our own resistance, we can see how listening to our babies' needs has helped us grow as individuals as well as parents. This approach could certainly never be called convenient, and no human being is capable of this kind of selfless giving all the time. Yet when done as much as humanly (and individually) possible, giving produces benefits beyond measure. The baby who is listened to grows into a toddler who is able to listen to the same degree to which his parents listened to him (not that he does so all the time, of course). By not forcing your power over him, you gain a smoother – though not easy – life with baby. On his own individual timetable he will be more and more able and willing to give you the lead when you need to take it, because he will have grown to trust you. Parents grow as people, learning how to give deeply of themselves, and baby grows as a person, learning he has the right to be heard and seen clearly. Both of these lessons help create healthy, mature adults.

Early on, the feelings experienced by parents of high-need children seem predominantly negative. Yet, we have noticed over the years of counselling these parents that their attitudes change to become mostly positive.

confident and comfortable

As you begin to see progress (and you will), your feelings will change from complete helplessness to realizing that you really do have a handle on your child's personality and needs. Those thousands of need-response moments have helped you know your child so deeply that you just know what you are doing is right, even if it is different from what your friends advise.

As parents again gain confidence, they feel increasingly comfortable (from the Latin for "with strength") caring for their high-need child. They seem to be more at ease handling their baby, responding spontaneously from inner convictions and using skills that have been sharpened over the months and years of learning, by trial and error, what works. As parents learn to comfort their child, they become more comfortable doing so.

I enjoyed my son's neediness. It forced me to sit and nurse all day. My major stress was the rude comments from in-laws about my "laziness" because the housework never got completely done and dinner was never prepared on time. What helped me was to realize that if you can create a

supportive frame of mind for yourself or with friends, having a high-need child doesn't feel like having a high-need child. It helped to arm myself with the facts and the benefits of my style of parenting so that nobody could shoot me down. In my heart I knew I was doing the very best for my family.

• • •

All of our children have been what many would call high-need: nursing every twenty minutes to two hours, needing to be held a lot, nursing at night for many months. However, we consider this normal behaviour, and with the help of the family bed, the baby sling, and La Leche League for support, we do not feel our children have been any "trouble". We have truly enjoyed all of our children. Perhaps the fact that I am the oldest of five children and a paediatric nurse and Dick is the oldest of four and a paediatrician helped us understand normal behaviour in children from the beginning and to know that each child is different. We have always made an effort to treat our children like we would like to be treated.

• • •

Once I started to educate myself, I felt better as a mother. I began to question the accepted, well meaning, and erroneous advice – even medical advice – I'd heard about babies and children. I found it was okay for me to hold him all the time and natural for me to feel anxious about leaving him. I learned to trust my instincts, and once I could do that, I could deal with my intense little baby. I'm happy to say that now I know. I know a baby wants to be in arms. That is natural. Anything else is desensitizing, I feel. I know it makes sense to sleep near your nursing baby. A mother gets so much more rest this way. I know it's okay to feel attached to my baby and trust my instincts. Now that Jay is older, I am more than ever convinced that if you meet the needs of a baby and youngster in the beginning, he will be much more secure and happy, and the mother-child relationship will be more positive later on. I know if I hadn't met my children's needs, they would be different people now.

proud

After realizing that many of those early, exhausting, high-need traits are blossoming into exciting personality features, you begin to feel less defensive or apologetic about having a "problem" child. You get over the unhelpful feeling that being different implies being less, and realize that in your child's case, being different means being more. She is more enthusiastic, more exciting, and more energetic, and has lots of other qualities that make her a hit with people. You will find yourself referring to your child in more positive terms, especially around those advisers, such as relatives, who early on could see only the negative.

I felt she would never leave my arms, but when she became two she began saying "my do it" a lot. I know this is a phrase that many mothers dread (because it takes five times as long to accomplish a simple task), but to the mother of a clingy baby, it is a joy. Now that Alex is suddenly absorbed in trying things herself, she is rapidly leaving behind many of her old baby needs, such as demanding to be carried everywhere and never leaving my lap. I must admit that there are times when I miss being the exclusive interest in her life, but when one of those moments arises, all I have to do is give her a big hug and she stops what she is doing and returns to me. Mostly, however, I am proud to see Alex growing into a happy, loving, self-confident little person, especially when I realize she has done it on her own – I have simply given her the support she needed.

vindicated

Even in those trying early months, when you doubt yourself and wonder if your in-laws are right in suggesting you let your baby cry, a voice inside tells you that what you are doing is right. Then, as your child's needs become easier to manage and you see your child's personality garden grow, the flowers begin to overshadow the weeds. Your child becomes your best argument that what you did was right.

My mother-in-law had been in our house about two hours when she began telling me point-blank I was doing everything wrong. She said we didn't need a Moses basket. Her babies went directly into their own cot in their own room, and I should not be feeding "that baby" in the bed. I should get up to feed him in a rocking chair in his own room so I wouldn't disturb my husband. She said I was feeding him way too often. (She had fed one of her babies on one

labelling

Labelling a child's behaviour can work for or against you. We've found "high-need child" to be generally a positive term, describing the signals a child gives and the level of parenting she needs. Positive labels both explain a child's behaviour and remind parents that their child is unique and special. Negative labels such as "difficult", "stubborn", and "manipulative" only serve to distance you from your child. They imply that your baby is intentionally trying to make her parents' life difficult. Labels run the risk of being judgmental, separating babies into "good" and "bad" categories. Be careful not to let a label become an excuse for a child's obnoxious behaviour, allowing you to sidestep the responsibility for reshaping this behaviour. Labels can easily become a substitute for discipline. If your two-year-old is being obnoxious and disruptive in the midst of a family gathering, don't excuse his behaviour with, "Oh, he's just high-need." Take charge and channel his behaviour in a more acceptable way. Remember, even high-need children must learn that other people also have needs. The following story is from two parents who looked past the labels to develop a deep understanding of their high-need child.

When we were tired and/or frustrated, we discovered how easy it was to slip into labelling Billy's behaviour as "difficult" or "intense" or "wilful". We also noticed that once a label was applied, it began to separate us from him and what he was trying to communicate. It put his behaviour in a nice, convenient category and served to protect us from our overwhelming feelings of helplessness and desperation. Labels obscured our view of the real child, who was simply expressing his needs in the only way he could.

When we found ourselves drifting into labelling Billy, we had to remind ourselves that his behaviour stemmed from a need or a feeling that had a right to exist. Labelling denied the complexity and value of his behaviour and boiled it down to terms that were too simplistic and almost always critical. Saying "Oh, he's just being difficult" not only assigns some very adult characteristics to a small child, but also negates anything that he is trying to communicate through his behaviour. I admit that it's still a challenge to maintain that image of the true child at 3am when he's struggling and twisting in my arms, but when I allow myself to see past the label, I am able to take a deep breath and once again see him for who he is and what he needs at that moment.

breast every four hours, and bottle-fed her other child.) She went on to preach that I was picking him up too often, and he was spoiled already. I would have to let him cry, and she wanted to know how soon I was going to wean him. I became so stressed at her trying to change my mothering style that on several occasions my milk supply diminished. I really needed her to take care of me and my house and let me take care of my baby.

It didn't end there. For two and a half years my in-laws openly criticized how I mothered my child. One time when I was staying with them while my husband was at a convention, I broke down and let my child cry. My father-in-law said he was a spoiled child and I had no control over him. He was controlling me. He would end up in the principal's office at school and in juvenile hall because I was ruining him. I finally confronted my mother-in-law in a letter and basically told her she had raised her children, now it was our turn to raise ours. And although we were doing things very differently from the way she did them, we were still good parents and our child was not a bad, spoiled child. He was just an active, high-need child. After the letter, the open criticism of me in front of my child stopped. As he got older, my in-laws mellowed a bit when they saw how bright and curious he is. They even commented, "He doesn't have that little mean streak that many children have."

connected

The most satisfying feeling you are likely to discover is the joy of being able to read your baby and respond intuitively to her cues and needs – and have her respond to yours. One of the most frequent comments we hear from mothers and fathers who have sensitively nurtured their high-need child is, "we're connected!" Because you never stop searching for answers and continue trying to find a style of parenting that works for both of you, you eventually get a handle on what makes your child tick and the level of parenting she needs to make family life run much more smoothly. There is great comfort that comes with knowing your baby and having a handle on her needs.

Seeing the results of hard work is rewarding, but experiencing the close relationship we share is the best payoff of all. Emily and I have gone through a lot together and we both know it. In doing so, we have formed an unbreakable bond of love and understanding, and that is what makes it all worthwhile.

• • •

What I appreciate most about your concept of high-need is that you celebrate this challenging temperament, rather than see it as a problem. When you described the characteristics of the high-need baby, I thought you had a secret camera in our house!

I feel Sam is completely normal. I certainly don't expect him to behave "better". But other people make comments or give me "that look" and ask if he is colicky. "He's high-maintenance", I say. With some of my more conventional friends, I sometimes feel defensive about Sam's personality and apologetic about my more "earth mother" caring style. Fortunately, I do have a circle of like-minded friends who support me!

I deeply appreciate knowing that someone else, particularly someone in the medical profession (known, in my experience, for its quick fixes), not only accepts but also celebrates the fussy baby's quirks and charms. Rather than trying to break Sam of his "bad habits", I feel free now to nurture him and to enjoy the special relationship we have and the cuddles that are my reward.

chapter 6

seventeen survival tips for parents of high-need children

You will survive. Your child will thrive. Life will go on. Still, it's hard to imagine even wanting to have another baby after you've held this one all day and been woken three or more times at night. It's hard to picture someone ever saying to you, "How blessed you are to have such an interesting child."

The journey from negative feelings to rewarding ones is a long uphill climb, but the payoff will come. Here are some survival tips that we discovered in parenting our high-need children and that other surviving parents have shared with us.

consider yourself

Mothers need mothering, too. All giving and no getting will wear thin. New mothers easily recognize themselves in this scenario: "My baby needs me so much that I don't even have time to take a shower." It's natural to put baby's needs first, but that doesn't mean you should always put your needs last. You can't parent a draining baby if you're drained. Next time you are on a plane, notice how the flight attendant demonstrates the proper use of oxygen: "Put on your oxygen mask before putting on your child's." If you are suffocating, you are no good to your child.

It helps to have a realistic appraisal of what you need in order to meet your baby's needs. Make a chart like the one opposite, and list the things you absolutely need for your well-being. Then make getting them a priority. Experiment with various activities that get your needs and baby's needs met at the same time. You will be amazed how much easier it is to care for your baby once you have cared for yourself.

I needed exercise and space. Yet my baby needed a lot of holding and motion. A half-hour morning walk met all these needs. I would wear him in a baby sling and take a walk along the most

Your Needs	Baby's Needs

peaceful path I could find. And each morning I would vary the route enough to keep it interesting for both of us. This is a great way to start the day. Besides being relaxing for me, the visual distractions of trees, flowers, traffic, kids, and people stimulated Matthew enough that he forgot to fuss.

allow baby some frustration

In your zeal to be a positive parent, it's tempting to keep giving until you give out. During the early months babies need a "yes-mother". Baby wants to feed; you oblige. Baby wants to be held; you hold her. Being unconditionally responsive is part of the parent-infant contract. Yet, such unconditional giving in the later months of baby care can develop into "martyr mothering" and actually interfere with your child's ability to begin developing a sense of self and a sense of competence. Worst of all, when done through gritted teeth (because you know deep down your constant giving is no longer appropriate for baby's age), responsive parenting deteriorates into resentful parenting. Once you know your limits, you will be motivated to find ways to get your baby to behave better, and your baby will soon get the message that life goes more smoothly with a mum who is happy. This will be especially true as your baby grows into toddlerhood and beyond.

Besides learning that if I wanted peace from her I needed to stay peaceful myself, toward the end of the first year it was better for her if I gradually eased off in responding to her cries. I will admit it was hard for me to make this transition from almost immediately responding to her cries to now frustrating her a little. I had to remain calm when I let her cry and not grow internally frantic. I learned to distract her calmly and to speak to her. I calmly communicated to her that I believed

too accepting?

Part of surviving life with a high-need child is to accept how your child is rather than how you wish he were. Yet there needs to be a balance to this acceptance. You don't need to simply roll over and play dead. You could resign yourself to the fact that you have a difficult child and you can't do anything about it. But this resigned acceptance will gradually wear out. It's easy with high-need babies to get into the downward spiral of expecting exasperating behaviour. You do have an obligation to shape your child's behaviour, to teach your child how to settle and control himself; otherwise the child runs wild and the family wears out.

she was okay and that I was still in charge of the situation. My being anxious communicated a sense of insecurity that would make her more upset and harder to calm down when I did pick her up.

• • •

I'm getting to know his limits and mine. There were days when I lost it; until I learned to put my three-year-old in his room, go to my room, and take a break. We both needed time out.

If your ten-month-old crawler gets himself into a corner and can't figure out how to make his way back out, his cries of frustration do not have to be answered immediately. He is secure enough now to be reassured by voice contact that you are on "standby". He may figure out how to solve his dilemma with a few words of encouragement from you. You certainly don't want to have to drop whatever it is you're doing and race to his rescue – unless, of course, his voice tells you he has hurt himself or he is frightened. (Even then, it's important for you to stay calm and quiet so that your peaceful presence can be a reassurance.) When a baby has been responded to quickly and calmly when he is younger, he will not have as much anxiety to deal with when he is older and you begin to allow, even encourage, a certain amount of frustration to enter his life. He needs these challenges so that he can continue in his development toward mature, healthy adulthood.

I needed to remain peaceful and calm when Libby was exploring and not interfere unless necessary. When she learned to crawl and climb, she was busy learning what her body could not do. I needed to be a peaceful presence, thus freeing her to concentrate on the task of learning. I was tempted to say things like, "Now, be careful" or "Watch out, don't fall", especially when she was crawling on the furniture. I noticed that my saying those things distracted Libby, forcing her to split her attention between the task at hand and tending to me. So, instead, I put myself where I could "spot" her and catch her if she was about to fall, and I calmly and quietly watched her. I did not want to interfere by looking or acting anxious.

This process often proves to be more difficult for the mother than for the baby. It is emotionally gratifying for most mothers to be loving and responsive to their babies. They struggle with this change toward their baby's growing independence because they don't understand how being "unresponsive" (albeit momentary and situational) could also be loving.

Here's another example from a mother who knew it was time to frustrate her older baby a bit so she could do something she wanted for herself:

The thing I really needed was to get Chris (my first) to the point where I could sit down at my sewing machine. Ohhhh, to me that was heaven! I found that once he was old enough to sit well, play on his own, and crawl around, I could steal as much as twenty or thirty minutes of sewing time at my machine. Sometimes it was a lot less than that. On teething days or sick days I wouldn't even try. But by gradually allowing him more "slack" to deal with the myriad mini-frustrations of the crawling stage, he learned that he could actually enjoy some mum-free time (and I certainly enjoyed my baby-free time). If he did come over to where I was working, often it was just to check in; or I would cheerfully encourage him to "go and get the ball" (or whatever) while I studiously focused on my sewing. He got the message it was okay for him to be on his own for a little while.

Many mothers of high-need toddlers can sympathize with what comes when they are pregnant with baby number two. It is quite a different situation to be pregnant when you already have an older child who is still quite demanding of you than it was to be pregnant the first time. Now when you want to spend some time doing prenatal exercises, you may find that you can include your toddler quite happily. If not, you can *calmly* let him know that this is mum's time to exercise and not to feed him. You *calmly* sit him on the couch where he can watch and firmly and sweetly insist he not pull on you anymore. You may have to exercise to a background of disgruntled noises, but if the noises become too irritating to you, you can give Jonathan the choice of looking at some books quietly or going to another room to fuss. You'll find that if you stay firm and cheerful (not at all angry), Jonathan will choose to stay and look at books, usually.

make sleep a priority

Sleep when your baby sleeps. Nap when your baby naps. It's tempting to "get things done" while your baby's napping. Resist that temptation and take a nap yourself. To keep your sanity in parenting a high-need child, you must make sleep and rest a priority. Martha has learned over the years that baby's sleep-time is pure gold – much too valuable to be spent washing dishes, dusting, or even cooking. Instead this precious recharge time was wisely put to use in ways that would make an eternal difference. In the early months the best way to spend it is with your baby sleeping right next to you (or even *on* you as some mothers of high-need babies learn to do to keep them sleeping longer). That way, even if you don't sleep, you are resting and bonding, getting your fill of that incredible baby smell and feasting your eyes on that darling face, so angelic in repose. As baby

Therapeutic Writing

When you've reached your wit's end, send your high-need child out to the park with father or a friend and sit down with your journal. Writing gives you the opportunity to examine your feelings about yourself, your parenting, and your child. It forces you to take inventory and proceed with what's working and discard what isn't. Journalizing helps you focus on the positive parts of your child rather than on the negative, and it enables you to see that life is getting better. Besides, when you're a grandmother, your journal will be a valuable gift if your child is blessed with a high-need baby. Pass your recorded wisdom on to the next generation.

Dear Dr Sears,
Thanks so much for encouraging me to write my story. You saved me a fortune in therapy!

gets older, you'll find that sitting nearby with a good book or some writing you want to do will be a rewarding way to spend this downtime. Think of it as school playtime. Only kids who are being punished for something have to spend their playtime *working*. Okay, well, once a month Martha used naptime to balance the chequebook, but only because it was impossible for her to do it without peace and quiet.

You will notice all these survival tips focus more on the mother than on the baby. When a mother of a high-need infant comes into our surgery for counselling, the first thing we ask is,

"How are you doing?" We have learned that if mother is doing well, in time baby will do well, too.

be positive

Your early feelings about having a high-need child may be so negative ("doesn't sleep", "won't settle", "uncuddly", "unpredictable", "stubborn") that you fail to see the flowers behind the weeds. The payoff in parenting a high-need child is that behind every apparent "negative" trait lies a positive one. Once you pull the weeds (yours and baby's), you see a flower blossom, sometimes so beautifully you forget that pile of weeds ever existed.

I have never met a high-need child who doesn't have one or more outstanding, positive character traits that, when found and nurtured, will later work to his or her advantage. The trick is to find them. It's so easy to let the negatives camouflage the positives. Sometimes you have to pull a lot of weeds to see the flowers bloom.

It helps to focus on what you like about your baby. "I'm glad he likes to feed so often; some of my friends had difficulty breast-feeding." "I'm happy she wants to be with me so much." "Thank heaven she's persistent. She knows what she wants and has the personality to get it."

I wasted so much time and energy wondering what problem my baby had and what I was doing wrong (because that's how my advisers made me feel). Once I started looking at the unique and positive qualities my baby had rather than at

how he inconvenienced me, mothering became much easier.

Take one day at a time. Don't dwell on the future. You can affect the future only by improving the present, anyway. It's normal to wonder if you'll ever get a full night's sleep, if you'll ever get a break, and if you'll ever have your partner all to yourself again. This is similar to the worry you had during pregnancy about whether you would ever have your old body back. Well, you eventually got your body back (or you will), but it was never quite the same. When we interview parents who have survived the early years of living with their high-need child, they nearly always report that this year is better than the previous one. The natural history of growth in parenting a high-need child is nearly always positive: the child becomes more manageable, and the parents become wiser. In fact, in interviews we've had with parents over the years, we nearly always see a gradual change in mindset from initial negativity about parenting a high-need child to overall positive feelings about the specialness of the child and the rewards to the family.

If you are a person who can't keep your mind off the future, consider this consoling thought: I suspect that many of the people who have done their part to make this world a better place to live were high-need children, raised in an environment that nurtured their needs rather than suppressed them.

Early on you will feel that nothing you are doing is working. This feeling won't last. You will always find some comforting technique that works, even if it works only once or twice and you then have to move on to experimenting with another technique (which also will work only for a little while). Rarely (if ever) do parents of high-need children complain that nothing works any of the time. And the more you try to comfort your baby, the more you hone your skills as a baby-comforter. You get better at the job. Consider this an opportunity as well as a trial. It's a parent-development process that you never would have experienced without a high-need baby. One mother lamented being exhausted from having to carry her baby all the time, but another mother accepted constant carrying with humour: "At least I'm getting my exercise."

be patient

We are rose lovers. Martha knows from experience that if she were to get impatient and try to unfold the rose petals by hand, the rose would look different in full blossom than if she were to patiently and lovingly wait for the petals to unfold themselves. The rose won't have the natural fullness it was meant to have. Just so, personalities don't change in a day. It may take months of hourly baby mellowing to notice progress.

We make allowances for his personality and temperament and give him time to catch up rather than pushing him to "straighten up" now. Sometimes I just resign myself to the fact that my child cries a lot and I can't always fix it, but I can at least be there.

focus on the "biggies"

As you learn to have more realistic expectations, be flexible, and, as surviving parents say, "go with the flow". It helps to save your energy and creativity for the "biggies", those rough edges in your child's personality that you simply can't tolerate and that you feel will later work to her disadvantage. Don't waste energy on the "smallies"; they will take care of themselves.

I worked for a Japanese company and learned a valuable parenting lesson: the Japanese don't waste time figuring out why a problem occurred or whom to blame; they focus on the solution. Devote your energy to what you can change and where you can make a difference, not to where you can't.

realize your child is unique

You may have entered parenthood with preconceived ideas of what children and babies are supposed to be like. Many of these assumptions come from being around other parents and their children. One of your earliest mind-set changes is to disregard what babies are "supposed" to act like, and focus on your baby, how your baby came wired, what your baby needs. As your child grows, you'll appreciate how important it is to see her as an individual.

What helped was for us to see our daughter as the intelligent person she is rather than trying to mould her to fit some standard model of babies. It also helped to change our expectations of her sleeping and nursing patterns and to concentrate on developing our own coping strategies. Around six months we began to see ourselves as being blessed with our high-need child instead of cursed. She taught us valuable parenting lessons that we never would have learned with a more complacent child. At first we were on the road

advice to friends and relatives

One of the hardest things for parents of high-need children is handling criticism from people they value. The parents are already struggling with feelings that their baby's personality is all their fault, that they are not good parents, and that their child is misunderstood. They are often made to feel embarrassed and apologetic for their child. You can help by being supportive. Talk about the qualities you like in the child. (Every child has some good points.) Don't offer sympathy – the child does not have a disease. Having high needs is not a "problem" or a "disorder"; it is a personality trait that is neither good nor bad; it's just there. When the parents are feeling down, pull them up. Be understanding, but you don't always have to join in the parents' misery. If the parents complain, "He's so draining", come back with "Yes, he certainly knows what he needs. And he's so enthusiastic." Hearing an uplifting comment from you may be just what the parents need. Parents who are doing their best to bring up a challenging child need your affirmation, not your criticism.

toward being controlling, manipulative parents, but Milly wouldn't have anything to do with that. We had to learn to be flexible and trust her to grow on her own terms, and be thankful for her lessons in life. She almost never wanted to be cuddly or sit and rock. She wanted us on our feet and moving constantly. Also, what worked for us was to take your advice "whatever works." What worked for Milly changed by the minute.

don't compare

This survival tip is a close cousin to the previous one. It's easy to label your child "bad" when he's the only one in the playgroup climbing on the kitchen counter while the others sit politely around the table having their snacks. It's easy to conclude that you're doing something wrong when your baby is, allegedly, the only one in the group who doesn't sleep through the night. New parents get their "norms" from the general parenting styles and child behaviour of whatever social group they're in. We live in a society in which being different is equated with being wrong. Not only is this faulty reasoning, but it will whittle away at whatever confidence you have left and undermine your perception of the uniqueness and value of your child. Comparing your parenting with others' will drive you nuts. You'll reinforce that negative nagging feeling that your child's behaviour is somehow your fault.

Avoiding the comparison trap frees you to look objectively at your child. You become less judgmental and more realistic. Your child came

wired differently from the one next door, not better, not worse – just differently. Every star shines a different light.

Although I love my child just as she is and try not to compare her to other children, it is very frustrating to see how much less demanding all my friends' children are. Her needs are so strong and my mothering of her has been so intense that sometimes I feel like we are from another planet. So many people just cannot understand her needs and the way I respond to them.

• • •

I was so tired of hearing the term "good baby". According to the norms of the neighbourhood, my baby wasn't "good". I then decided that a baby is "good" when he cries and lets you know what he needs. (In other words, all babies are "good".) That really put a new perspective on fussy babies for me. They cry more because they need more.

• • •

My advice to parents is that if you had a sick child, you would give that child the care that she needed; so if you have a high-need child, give her the extra attention she needs. She needs it for a reason.

• • •

Once I learned that she has high needs for a developmental reason, it was easier for me to respond accordingly.

get out

Home to a child is where mother is. The open space of a park or playground can release a tenacious child and relax a tense parent.

The biggest help I've found is being outside. We now have a large garden, and my parents have filled it with toys. This is a large factor in keeping my sanity. Being able to just sit while my children burn off all of their energy is truly a blessing.

if you resent it, change it

The key to surviving and thriving with a high-need child is to keep working until you find a parenting style that meets the needs of your child but at the same time does not exceed your desire or ability to give. You will have to stretch yourself, but not until you snap. In counselling parents of high-need children, a key question that we have found helpful in deciding when parents need to change what they are doing is, "Do you resent what's going on?" "Are you becoming increasingly resentful of your style of parenting?" If the answer is yes, you need to make a change. Continuing to tough it out in a style of parenting that may be working for your baby but is not working for you will make you become angry and increasingly resentful of your baby. Everyone resents parenting at times. It's a difficult, stress-filled job. Determine what you can change and what you can't; but, above all, learn how not to resent what you are doing.

Getting past this point of resentment sometimes means that you must change what you're doing or change your understanding of your child. Sometimes it means you must change your own attitude. Most situations call for adjustments in all three areas. Here's an example: your six-month-old awakens daily at 6:15am raring to go and demanding playmates. You are a night person, hate getting up at dawn, and like to wake up slowly, preferably with a cup of coffee and the paper. You're sleep-deprived already from nighttime feeding, and you really resent your baby's intrusions into your waking habits. What do you do? Here are three suggestions for handling your dilemma:

1. Change what you're doing. If possible, have dad get up with baby so that you can sleep another half-hour or forty-five minutes. Or, gradually shift baby's bedtime to a later hour so that he'll sleep longer in the morning.
2. Change your understanding of your child. At six months, he may be ready to play by himself first thing in the morning. Surround him with interesting toys reserved only for morning play on the kitchen floor while you eat your toast and read the paper. If he fusses, help him out a bit and then go back to your paper for a few more minutes. He'll survive.
3. Change your attitude. Morning may not be your favourite time of the day, but it can be a quiet, peaceful time. Wake up to relaxing music. Make some herbal tea or eat last night's pasta for breakfast. And remember that these special mornings with your baby will last only a short time. Soon you'll have to get up early to get your children ready for school.

My baby constantly demands to be held and walked, and has to be entertained virtually at all times. I can't leave her alone for a minute. I even have to take her to the bathroom with me. When she does sleep, I'm torn between whether I should get some rest myself or try to get something done around the house. I feel I should not be separated from this child day or night. Sometimes (but not very often) I have to let her cry because I'm on the verge of losing it, and then I feel guilty because I know she wants me but I've got to get away from her. I wish there were support groups for people with babies like this, but I probably couldn't attend anyway because my daughter cries even when we're riding in the car. I can't go anywhere! I love this child and I hope I don't sound selfish when I say "WHAT ABOUT ME?" I have become a slave to this baby. Anything I want or need is not important. When I read that the two of you have eight children I said, "These people have lost their minds." My husband works twelve- to fourteen-hour shifts, so he's not here a lot of the time. (Besides, he can't get her to stop crying the way I can.) I'm afraid to leave her with anyone because I'm honestly afraid she will get neglected or, even worse, shaken by someone who doesn't know her like I do. I feel better just writing all this down. I guess it's like therapy. I also know I will survive this, and the only real cure is time. She will grow and this will all be in the past someday.

We hope this mother will read Chapter 7, "Mother Burnout".

get help

The earlier you realize that in parenting a high-need child you will need outside help, the better you will survive. Choose your allies carefully. Unless they have a high-need child, they may have difficulty empathizing with you. Surround yourself with like-minded parents. Join a high-need support group, or start your own.

Friends and relatives who have watched us mother Katie over the past two years have offered us love and support, despite the fact they do not always understand. When I hear wonderful compliments like, "You have done so well with such a difficult baby" and, "You and Katie are an inspiration to me when I am having a bad day with my baby", I feel like all the hard work is worth it. We need someone to tell us that we are doing something right. It really helps to hear positive comments from other people, even though I can see for myself where my mothering efforts are paying off.

• • •

Finding a support group and supportive friends has helped me to cope with our fussy baby. It is so important to be able to complain to understanding people about the baby you love so dearly. Early on I learned whom to complain to. La Leche League mums were unmatched in their understanding of mothering a fussy baby. Their support has been a real confidence-booster. The support group that has given me the most satisfaction in my mothering accomplishments is our playgroup. Some mothers in it were initially

support groups

When your misery needs company, form a "high-need child" support group. Surrounding yourself with other parents who share your plight and your point of view helps you see the specialness of your child. You will also get some valuable child-management tips from experienced parents. Other parents in your support group will be willing to listen to your story over and over, and without judgment. You don't have to fear that you are "messing up" in front of them, because the rest of the group members are also struggling to find their way in managing a high-need child.

I posted some flyers in shops and at my GP's surgery and started a support group. We met at a park two to four times a month and used *the phone for in-between support. The upside was seeing other difficult children and hearing their mums' war stories. The downside was trying to get everyone there because of these unpredictable children. ("Unpredictable" was Julia's middle name. Her mood was inconsistent and changed without apparent reason. I just never knew what kind of day we were going to have.) We discussed survival tips and management strategies (when we weren't keeping our difficult children from killing each other). It helped to know that there were other people out there struggling just as I was. I soon found that local GPs were referring their high-need patients to our support group. Perhaps these doctors were just as frustrated as we were.*

sceptical of my reports of Emily's fussiness. When they got to know us, they began to agree that my intensive mothering was the only way to go with my baby. A few have even changed their own parenting skills. One mother has told me that if I can get through each day with Emily, she knows she can make it through the day with her kids.

• • •

One day when my baby was one month old, I was talking to my mother on the phone and I said, "Mum, I've been crying for two days and I can't stop, and I'm getting scared." Mum came right over. We had a talk, and she said, "Donna, it's *okay to feel resentful that your life has been turned upside down by this precious little baby girl." I said, "That's exactly how I feel. I don't resent her, but I resent the fact that I have no life anymore. I'm trying to keep her content, and I don't seem to be able to succeed at that." I felt very isolated and depressed. Mum said, "I'll take Lauren tonight, and you and Michael go out for dinner. Lauren wouldn't take a bottle, so I showed Mum how to use a medicine cup to give her breast milk in case she got hungry. I fed her before we left, tanked her up, then left her with my mum for a couple of hours while Michael and I went out to dinner.*

job-share

The person who shared in the conception must also share in the care of the child. Trying to practise attachment parenting without your partner's help can wear you out if you don't have extended family to help. Share the job, share the joy. A giving mother and an involved father is a win-win-win situation: you gain much-needed help; your partner gets closer to his child and develops creative fathering techniques; and your child gets used to the variety of comforting techniques that father can provide.

Part of the problem was that my husband was working long hours. I was the only one home with Suzanne for the majority of the time. And I felt I needed to keep her quiet at night so my husband could get his much-needed sleep because of the "high-need business" he was in. I didn't want him to fall asleep on the motorway during his hour-long drive to work. But I realized I was wearing out. One night David and I went out to dinner. As we talked, we realized that while I was trying to keep him from the frustration of having a high-need, colicky baby because I was concerned about his safety driving and the long hours he was working, he was actually wanting to be involved and wanting to get up and relieve me at night, but didn't want to displace my role as the mother. At that point we decided it was time to work together as a team, and we'd either take shifts during the nighttime hours or we'd just be up together in the middle of the night. I would get up and feed her or just pull her close to me in bed and feed her. If she wouldn't fall asleep from that,

David would take her and walk with her. Sometimes when we were up together, it gave us a chance to share our feelings about having a high-need baby and how this was affecting our feelings for each other. We realized we had been growing apart, but now that we began sharing our baby's care, all three of us grew back together.

• • •

Out of necessity and because of the intense physical and emotional demands of a high-need newborn, we developed a real sense of balance in our relationship. I would get tired, and Jim would take over. He would get discouraged, and I would feel hopeful. It allowed us to become acutely aware of our own limitations and to develop our own particular strengths in soothing Karen. These strengths were added to our colic "bag of tricks" and brought out as the situation warranted. We learned when to ask for help and when to take over – when Karen needed mum and when she wanted dad.

Two months after Karen was born, we went to a reunion of our childbirth class. This day proved to be a real learning experience for us all. At one point, Karen indicated that she was sleepy. Since she was not a baby who would simply doze off when she was tired, Jim took her in his big arms and bounced her down to sleep. When he got too hot from holding her, he would pass Karen to me. I would take her and bounce her while he ate. Then he would take her back while I ate. It was the beginning of our own version of the "colic dance". It's a dance we continue to this very day.

We remember feeling somewhat scrutinized, as if all the other parents' eyes were on us. But instead of feeling unsure, we gained confidence that day, not only in our ability to help Karen and make her feel safe and comfortable in any environment, but also in our ability to work as a team. That, too, continues to be an important and valued characteristic of our family.

plan ahead

Learn to anticipate your child's needs, and avoid, as much as possible, situations that set you up for conflicts. If your baby is a late-afternoon fusser, stay clear of supermarkets during those hours. After the first few months, you will know at which times of the day your child's moods are easier to manage, and you can then structure your day accordingly. Mornings are usually magnificent for high-need babies and their somewhat rested parents. That may be your so-called quality time. Toward the end of the day is usually comfort time, the 4:00 to 8:00pm "happy hours" when babies are usually the least manageable. Try to avoid unsettling activities during those hours and concentrate on meeting your baby's needs. (See the related discussion of anticipating your baby's pre-cry signals, page 53.)

Taking him anywhere had to be planned in advance. Before going out, I would do an imaginary run-through of where we were going, what we were going to do, what behaviour I could expect of him, and how I could best adjust my agenda to keep us both happy. I had a backup game plan if things didn't go well. Before I could do this, I had to work hard to overcome the influence of outside pressures that I was spoiling him, letting him manipulate me, or that my life was becoming too child-centred. Once I learned to rearrange my life around my child's needs and personality, we were both much more relaxed. We take into account our child when planning our activities. We take into account his needs and ours. We've learned to be flexible and leave spaces of time in our schedule for a change of plans.

● ● ●

During the first three months, Jonathan was so fussy, I gave up trying to cook dinner between 5:00 and 7:00pm. I would just wait until my partner got home or I would cook earlier in the day when my baby was asleep. I also gave up trying to keep a neat, tidy house. I tend to be a neat freak. I like things orderly and under control, but I realized that if I focused too much on housework I was going to miss out on the fun of playing with my baby.

The ability to plan and anticipate is learned from one's parents. It is a valuable life skill for everyone, not just for parents. It implies a certain level of personal discipline so that you don't have to "fly by the seat of your pants" or cope with the pressure of rushing around at the last minute. Having a high-need child will make very clear to you whether you anticipate well or not. With this skill, you'll avoid putting either yourself or your child into impossible situations. People who have never learned to make realistic plans may need professional help to learn this skill as adults.

take the long view

Consider that you're into parenting for a lifetime. Shaping a child's behaviour is a gradual process. You will not see daily change. Coping with slow improvement may be especially difficult if you are a person used to quick fixes. Remember, you are dealing with a person, not a machine.

I can't choose my child's temperament, but I can influence its outcome.

• • •

I learned to judge developmental progress on a long-term basis. I stopped asking myself if Jonathan was doing better this week than last week. Instead I compared this year's behaviour to last year's. It helped me a lot, because I could see good progress over the long term, even when we were having a rough week.

• • •

The turning point was when a friend convinced me that my baby was only a baby a short time, and she would only be a tiny infant once, and the decisions I made and still make will affect her as she grows.

• • •

My partner and I feel that the amount of time we spend with our baby in our arms not only builds strength in our bodies but also helps to build strength in our family.

get behind the eyes of your child

Throughout your parenting career there will be thousands of situations that test your composure. Your toddler throws a fit at playgroup when you announce it's time to go. Your child spills juice all over her shirt when you're already late for an appointment. The first thought that flashes through your mind is likely to be, "How inconvenient for me." But beware; these initial adult-centred thoughts can trigger a whole chain of events that only make things worse.

At three, our Lauren had an especially quick trigger, and we learned that she was unreachable once she was flooded with anger. The thing that most set her off was getting an angry reaction from one of us. This caused us to consider carefully controlling our emotions when all we would achieve otherwise was to send Lauren into a tailspin.

Of course, even now it never is worth it to get angry with Lauren (but we don't always remember this in time to salvage a situation). She, with her high sensitivity to an insult, has taught us not to insult her. We've learned to say calmly, "Oops, a spill. Let's wipe it up." (She's very good at cleaning up.) And we are getting better at staying calm.

Instead of getting stuck in the rut of thinking how aggravating or inconvenient a situation is, get into the mind of your child and consider the effects of the situation on him. This approach is not only less upsetting to the child, it's less

making major changes

High-need children are slow to adapt to major changes in family life. Moving is one such change. Young infants usually don't have a problem because to them home is where mummy is, even though mummy's in a new house. With older children you can smooth the process by helping your child with the transition. Prepare the child for the move by emphasizing the positive – new friends, his own room, perhaps a larger garden to play in or a park nearby. Let him help you prepare for the move and get the new house ready. Pack up his things last and unpack them first. Expect your child to show behaviour swings during a move because of the stresses you will naturally undergo. The more quickly you settle into a new routine, the more quickly your child's behaviour will return to normal.

distressing for you. One day I watched the mother of an accident-prone, high-need two-year-old handle an upsetting situation. The child dropped the milk carton from the refrigerator shelf and the milk spilled all over the floor. The mother knelt next to the child, looked at the mess, and turned to her child empathically. For a few seconds she didn't say anything. And then I watched how the child willingly helped the mother mop up the mess. After the job was done, neither mother nor child was upset, and the day went on with no energy lost. I asked the mother why this potentially messy situation turned out so positively. She volunteered, "Right

after Beth spilled the milk, I asked myself, if I were Beth, what would I want my mother to say?" This mother's first impulse was to project herself into the mind of her child, which triggered a whole chain of empathic and appropriate responses, and saved a lot of mental wear and tear on everyone. To do this on a consistent basis, you will need to be taking good care of yourself – avoiding too much stress, eating right, sleeping enough, keeping balance in your life emotionally and physically. Needless to say, this doesn't always happen, and then both of you pay the price.

As a two-year-old, our Matthew was (as he still is) a very focused child. Scooping him up from play without warning simply because of a grown-up agenda was certain to invite a tantrum. Though it was at times inconvenient, Martha realized that Matthew's ability to concentrate and focus on his play was a valuable trait, useful in later life. So, instead of expecting Matthew to switch from his agenda to hers, she gave Matthew a warning a few minutes before it was time to leave, giving him time to make the transition. Then she helped him remove himself from what he was doing: "Matthew, say bye-bye to the trucks, bye-bye to the cars, bye-bye to the toys, bye-bye to your friends …" This gave Matthew a chance to leave his activity gradually and with a sense of closure. (And remember, in order for this to happen, Martha had to have enough self-discipline to start early and allow enough time, so that there would be no pressure-filled deadlines for leaving.) We also used this "saying bye-bye to everyone (and everything) in the room" approach in making the transition to going to bed. Considering the child's feelings first instead of yours is not a threat to your authority or control; it's good strategy in all human relationships.

it's no one's fault

Having a high-need baby is really a no-fault situation. Your baby is the way she is, and you are the way you are. The key is to get your personalities to mesh rather than clash.

The biggest improvement in her behaviour happened at the same time I was able to accept her as she was, and not as something that I had to fix or that was my fault.

study your child

You must become an expert on your child; no one else will. There is no such thing as a parenting expert, only parents who have a lot of experience and who have learned, through years of trial and error, what works for them. Yet, remember, their experience is gleaned from parenting their own children and may not apply to your family. Professionals learn by interaction with lots of parents and children. Most are simply opinion givers, and you will find some opinions more useful than others. Unlike the impression conveyed by popular magazine articles, parenting a high-need child requires more than a list of "Ten Easy Ways to Parent". You

must individualize your parenting style. This comes only as a result of studying your child moment by moment, learning to read her body language, and anticipating her moods and needs so that you can be one step ahead of your child. You become an encourager who shapes your child's personality, a facilitator who makes it easier for the child to get through difficult times, and an organizer who makes it possible for your child to succeed without tantrums. While professional counselling has its place, you may discover that few advisers truly understand high-need children – unless, of course, they have raised one.

At two months of age, Laura continues to teach us, and we continue to be good students. We do not yet speak each other's language, but we've progressed day-to-day as we learn a language based on intuition, trust, and a profound respect for each other.

the high-need parent

High-need children and parents need:

- *more* understanding
- *more* encouragement
- *more* help
- *less* criticism

In fact, "high-need" not only describes the child, it describes the *relationship* between parents and child. "High-need family" says it all.

handling criticism

Having a high-need child can make you an easy target for critics. The hardest thing is having others think that by trying to meet your child's needs you have created them, and by being sensitive to them you're making them worse. To protect yourself and your child from unwanted and unhelpful advice, try these suggestions:

Keep your complaints private
Going public with your complaints exposes you to critics. Choose carefully to whom you gripe. Don't ask questions you don't want answered. If your misery must have company, seek the ear of like-minded friends who share your parenting philosophy, preferably ones who are also parenting a high-need child.

Protect yourself
If your critics conclude you are withering away, they will feel compelled to water you with advice. They may assume that your baby is a burden to you and what you really need is a break from your baby. Set the record straight: "Actually, I love having my baby with me all the time." In effect, you are conveying, "I'm okay, I don't need your help with the baby, thank you." Of course, if there are other kinds of help you need – with the dishes, opening a door – now may be a good time to ask. When critics suggest that your parenting style is spoiling your baby, tell them, "Babies can't be spoiled … only nurtured" or "Babies, like food, only get spoiled if they are left unattended on a shelf."

Shield your child
It's easy for your child's self-image to be affected by comments from friends and relatives. Don't let negative vibrations rub off on your child. If you're invited to a home where you know critics are going to give your child a "Why aren't you like the other children?" message, don't go. Don't discuss your child's challenges within his hearing.

I think my child thinks he's bad, and that breaks my heart. I'm certain he sensed my doubts and picked up on the criticism of the other family members who thought he was just a bad boy. I reassure him he's not bad. He's got spirit and chutzpah. When he was three years old he told my auntie, "I'm bad, aren't I?" This has been particularly difficult because our second child has a completely different temperament and seems to be so "good".

Be positive
Friends and relatives will pick up on how you assess your own child. If you are negative, complaining, and seem overwhelmed by your high-need child, expect friends to react the same way. But, if you seem excited and proud to have this energetic child, they will be impressed with her positive qualities rather

than regarding her as your "problem child". If a critic pronounces, "My, she is obstinate", come back with "Yes, she's very persistent." When the critic says, "He's so boisterous", come back with "He has a lot of enthusiasm."

Since Emily does not handle being away from me well at all, my partner and I made a decision that we will not leave her again until she is old enough to understand what is going on. She tends to fuss when she is with, or around, people she doesn't see on a regular basis, and people act like there is something the matter with her. They say things like, "Oh, Molly, you've got to get away from her." But I don't want to get away from her! My mother was passing around my eight-month-old niece the other day, and as the baby went from person to person without a sound, my mother said, "Isn't she a good baby?" I feel that Emily is a good baby, too, even though she is a high-need baby. During a recent doctor visit, my mother-in-law went along to watch Emily while I was seeing the doctor. Afterward she said something that was music to my ears: "What a well-adjusted, happy child."

Consider where the source got her parenting info

Your mother really does have your best interests and those of her grandchild at heart, but she raised you in an era when routines, bottle-feeding, cots, playpens, smacking, and fear of spoiling were standard. Naturally, her

views on child rearing will differ from yours. Accept this. Nothing divides friends and relatives like differences of opinion on raising kids. Pick out those childcare practices that you and your mother agree on, and keep the conversation centred on those; for the rest, simply agree to disagree.

My worst problem has been dealing with outside pressure, criticism, and intolerance of my parenting style – especially from my mother, who can actually be cruel and will not let things go. She insists I have made things harder for my son by breast-feeding and not using a playpen. I try hard to avoid the sleeping arrangement subject with her, because she thinks I should be ashamed of myself for not putting Alan in a cot at night; but she tends to bring it up in search of an argument. She is beginning to pressure me to wean him; she has no conception of baby-led weaning and will be horrified when she hears about my plans to let him wean himself. She really enjoys her grandson (although sometimes at my expense), and I don't want to take that away from her, but I have considered moving far away.

• • •

The greatest challenge I have found has not been meeting the needs of my child, but responding to criticisms of our parenting style. Even our family doctor, who was wonderful throughout our pregnancy, has expressed doubts about our approach. It's as if they believe our attentiveness has caused his personality, rather than the other way around.

Surround yourself with encouragers, not critics. Don't feel you have to defend your child or explain your parenting styles to everyone. Your child will have many critics, but only one set of parents who know what is best. Eventually, your child will become the living proof that what you have done is right. As your critics see your child blossom, they will realize that your heart did indeed lead you to the right way of parenting that child. A few may even be glad that you didn't take their advice.

As you grow in your knowledge of your child, you will find yourself becoming increasingly confident about the value of your own intuition; yet this will be a slow process, based on hundreds of moment-by-moment, trial-and-error decisions. Once you get in sync with your child, you will be able to stop relying on outside advice and trust yourself.

My most important advice for other parents of high-need children is this: listen to your instinct and listen to your baby. I have always assumed that Katie cried or fussed for a reason, even if I couldn't figure out what it was. The more I followed her cues and my own feelings and observations (instead of others' advice), the easier it became to promptly meet her needs, help her feel content, and become more self-confident as a mother.

Have confidence in yourself and in your parenting. This will be your best survival guide.

chapter 7

mother burnout

Having our first high-need child introduced us to the problem of mother burnout. Caring for Hayden's high needs fanned the flames of Martha's deep commitment to mothering. And, as often happens when something is on fire, burnout was not far behind.

martha's experience

As a mother of eight, I have been in and out of burnout more often than I care to remember. I have learned a lot about how it happens, how to get out of it, and, more recently, how to keep it from happening. Much of what I have learned has come through some very special friends, mothers who have been there and learned the hard way that they must take care of themselves in order to take care of their children. I've also learned from some very special support groups – La Leche League groups I've been in and led over the past seventeen years, a women's support group devoted to learning a better way of living, and a number of church prayer groups that have helped me learn about spiritual nourishment.

Burnout is, to me, the most important hurdle mothers have to face. If they succeed in overcoming it, mastering it, and preventing it, they succeed as mothers. If they fall victim to it and never or rarely come out of it, they will have a very unfortunate life and a very disadvantaged family. I believe that much of what I've experienced was passed down to me by several generations of burned-out mothers. One of my main goals in my own life has been to break the cycle of damaged emotions and relationships caused by burnout so that my own children, and especially my daughters, experience less struggle.

So just what is mother burnout? The term defies a one-sentence definition, but a good place to start would be to say that mother burnout is a condition in which a mother feels overwhelmed with her circumstances, with little or no reserves available to cope with the demands on her time, her energy, her whole being – physical, mental, emotional, and spiritual. There are degrees of mother burnout, ranging from the state you find yourself in when you've been up all night with a sick child and you have no one to help you the next day to the extreme of postpartum psychosis, which could be termed "mother meltdown". No matter what degree of burnout a mother is experiencing, she needs help on all levels – physical, mental, emotional, and spiritual.

My friend Gina has been studying mother burnout for ten years (her oldest child is ten!). She has mastered the art of recognizing, treating, and preventing it, and has generously taught what she has learned to any mother who has asked her for help, including me. She developed a pamphlet, a teaching tool to use in helping mothers recognize, treat, and prevent burnout in themselves. Here is a list she compiled from mothers stating how they feel when they are burned out.

- I feel overwhelmed.
- Every little thing annoys me.
- I explode over meaningless incidents.
- I need to escape.
- I feel out of control.
- I am afraid I will hurt my baby.
- I feel like hitting my older kids.
- I feel like screaming.
- I feel like crying all the time.
- I feel angry, frustrated.
- I resent the baby and his needs.
- I feel guilty for resenting this little baby.
- I feel jealous of my baby, who's getting more of her needs met than I am.
- I feel guilty for how badly I treat my partner and older kids.
- I feel guilty for yelling so much.

- Nothing is funny anymore.
- I feel as if I can't get up in the morning.
- I feel jealous of my partner leaving the house every day.
- It's too much to handle when even little things go wrong.
- My partner and kids can't do anything right.
- I feel exhausted.
- I feel like I will fall over if I close my eyes.
- I feel exhausted even when I get enough sleep.
- I can't sleep even though I feel exhausted.
- I want to sleep all the time.
- I don't want to eat and I am losing weight.
- I eat all day long and gain weight.
- I spend too much money.
- I pinch pennies unnecessarily.
- I crave food or drinks or substances that are not healthy for me and baby.
- I feel that everything needs to be just so.
- I feel I need to be babied for a change.
- I feel that I can't do anything right.

what fuels mother burnout?

To remedy a problem it is important to identify its causes; otherwise the problem will never really be dealt with. We may feel relief from time to time as circumstances wax and wane; but the problem will always be there the next week, the next day, even the next hour (or minute). I didn't begin to get a handle on my burnout until I took a look at what was causing it. (By the way, every mother experiences these problems at one time or another. It's how we learn to respond to them that matters.) These are the causes of burnout:

another baby? – maybe

In the first year or two of living with a high-need baby, having another will be the furthest thought from your mind; yet normal biological urges tend to erase the weeks and months of sleepless nights and constant holding. It's normal to start yearning for another infant sometime during your child's second year. While how far apart to space children is a highly personal decision, in general, parents of high-need children tend to wait at least three years before having another child. The child's need for high maintenance, while it never completely goes away, certainly lessens around the third birthday, when many high-need children develop an unexpected desire for independence and an "I do it myself" attitude. A high-need child who got his needs well met when he was younger will have less difficulty seeing his new sibling get what he used to get. He may occasionally make noises about wanting what baby has (and he certainly will need reassurances that he is still very important to you), but he'll also be ready to move on to a relationship with dad that will balance out what he no longer receives from mum.

Many mothers of high-need children have found they were unable to conceive for three to four years after their high-need child was born, as if both their body and their subconscious confirmed they weren't ready for the undertaking. This was true for Martha. We used to joke about how Hayden put off having a new sibling come along until she was ready to share Martha. (Erin was born when Hayden was four and a half, though we had made no attempt to avoid conception.) Our other children, after the first two, were spaced three years apart because of the natural break in fertility that extended breast-feeding gave us. Actually, pregnancy was held off, probably not so much by Hayden's high-need behaviour as by Martha's subconscious realization that she was not ready to have another baby.

Trying to do too much, too soon. Often the most physically demanding period in the life of a mother is when her baby is a newborn. She's just come through the most demanding hours (or days) of her life, only to launch into a series of physical exertions that can quickly become over-exertions. That is, unless she lives in one of those enlightened cultures that provide a doula (servant) to be at her side continuously, helping her provide comfort and nourishment for her baby by doing everything for her that she needs done, for as long as she needs it. If she is such an honoured woman, she's probably not reading this book!

In cultures that hold mothering in esteem, there are no doubts that every woman is physically capable of bearing and nurturing children, yet she does not do it on her own. She would think it is crazy to have to read a book to learn how to be a mother. Sadly, our culture tells women that we are not physically competent to do what we are born to do, and we have lost much of our intuition. A woman in our culture is expected to do it on her own, and she struggles with loss of sleep, energy expenditure in making milk, hormones readjusting, delayed meals, missed meals (if she's not taking care of herself), extra nutritional needs, extra laundry, needing to be on her feet so much more with a high-need baby, plus all the other physical demands of "life going on", depending on the needs of any other children she may have. This alone would be enough to push a healthy woman who had an "easy" birth close to burnout. If the birth was physically traumatic in any way, she must add healing to the list.

Worry. Worry can zap a major portion of a mother's energy and leave her feeling burned out. There are so many possible worries in the day of the mother of a newborn. Will she be a good mother? Can she even *do* this? What *is* a good mother? Why is her mate suddenly so tense? What is she not doing that he needs? (This worry is probably more correctly placed in the category of wife burnout, but it has negative effects on mothering, too.) If baby wakes up more often than she expects, she wonders if something is wrong. If baby sleeps more than she expects, she wonders if something is wrong. Why is baby squirming and fussing at the breast so much today? When baby cries in that certain way, she panics because she doesn't know if what she did yesterday to help him will work today. Mothers spend their days thinking for

feeling touched out?

Human touch is probably the most powerful way to affect another human being. Without touch, or enough of it, babies would die. Can there be too much of a good thing? Can a mother be in such constant touch with her baby that she does not seek out touch from her mate? Can even this baby/toddler touch be more than she ever bargained for and something she looks forward to being finished with? Many of us, in our Western culture, experience these feelings as a result of being touch-deprived in infancy – a by-product of experts telling our mothers to "put that baby down". The good news is that you can actually benefit from all this touch time. Give yourself permission to enjoy (savour!) touching, holding, and wearing your baby. At the same time as you ensure your baby won't be touch-deprived, you'll also be getting in some makeup touch time for yourself. Don't worry about overdoing it. A baby who gets enough touching will squirm free, wriggle down, and push you away when he's ready. Then all you have to do is let your toddler go (it will happen!) and surprise your mate with your new-found craving for touch.

baby. Unless they are very competent mothers there are lots of opportunities to worry, and that's just the beginning. What about when he's a crawler, a toddler, a preschooler …? What will the world be like in twenty years? The list of possible worries grows exponentially. No wonder worry can wear us out!

Mothering beyond one's personal resources. No matter how much we know or how our hearts lead us, we still tend to mother "from our gut". When push comes to shove, we tend to do what has been done to us. If we were not nurtured or given to as infants, we may lack the emotional resources for the task of nurturing and giving freely to our own babies. No matter how deeply a mother believes her baby needs to be held or how much she wants to hold her, she still may feel she's giving (and getting) too much touching if she holds her baby much of the day. (This may affect how she regards her mate, too.) Possibly, way back when this mother was an infant, the experts or an interfering grandma advised *her* mother to "put that baby down" or said, "See, she's spoiled! She stopped crying the instant you picked her up." Mothers may believe in nurturing, but it doesn't always *feel* good.

Even with a background of having been well nurtured, mothers may find they are running on empty when circumstances draw too heavily from their emotional tanks. Even the most centred of mothers can be pushed past her resources. For some, it takes very little: a missed shower or a late lunch. For others, it takes a great deal: a move or job loss, an illness or death in the family, *and* a missed shower or a late lunch. In either case, the burned-out feeling is just as real.

A build-up of resentment due to unmet expectations. Every day, all day, we have expectations, conscious and unconscious. I expect my hair to lie a certain way, this chair to feel a certain way underneath me, my partner to come home at a certain time, the floor to be clean and the dishes washed. When our expectations are unmet, we often choose to resent it. Built-up resentment can wear a mother out faster and more thoroughly than physical overexertion. Mothering fills the day with expectations that go unmet. My baby should be taking longer naps, shorter naps, more naps, fewer naps. I should be able to eat my food when it's hot with no interruption. I should be, feel, or look in shape by now. Other people should accept and support what I am doing as a mother. You could fill a book with all the expectations we have in just one day.

what to do about it

There are ways you can deal with each of these causes of burnout. You can pull yourself out of ordinary burnouts using the following insights along with things you learn on your own and from others in your support system. More persistent burnout is severe depression and may include recurring thoughts of suicide or an inability to function during the day or sleep at night. For this you probably need professional help, in which case the following can tide you over until you can find it.

Helpful hints for physical strength. Do whatever it takes to get the rest and sleep you need. In the first few months with baby, never let housework and errands rob you of rest. Don't underestimate the devastating effects of continuous, serious sleep deprivation on your ability to mother. Get help from family, friends, neighbours, church; hire a doula or a teenager.

"my partner works too much"

If your partner works too much, you probably won't be able to change that. He may eventually figure out that this is a problem and gradually make some changes himself. But until that happens, you can be happy yourself and find additional support systems to fill the gap. After all, just because he has chosen to be a workaholic doesn't mean you have to be miserable yourself and give your children an unhappy mother. You'll need to say to yourself, "He's doing what he has to do" (and, after all, he does have to earn a living and may be busy finding his identity at this stage in his maturity from the work he does). You can rise above the expectations you have had that he will be available frequently to help you. When he is home, make the most of the time you have together by being positive and undemanding. That doesn't mean you never let him know what needs doing, but you do it politely and graciously. For example, "Would you please take out the rubbish?" instead of "This rubbish is driving me crazy. You never even see it!" Then find ways to nurture yourself and get the support you need from friends and from doing what keeps you peaceful and happy.

Remember to move at a slower pace and do only what contributes to keeping up your milk supply. (A low milk supply will make baby fussy.) Watch your fluid intake, rest when you need rest, and keep your feet up a lot. Do some relaxation exercises, like deep breathing and stretching, especially when your muscles are tense. It helps to remember that physical work you don't enjoy (resent) is more likely to cause you aches and pains, so keep a conscious check on your attitude. If you're not enjoying your baby (hard work and all), find out why.

Keep an eye on your own physical health. Emotions can be affected by problems in your body, and your body can be affected by your emotions. See a doctor who is able to treat the whole person, body and soul, if you are feeling run-down physically, especially if you get sick a lot. A weakened immune system can open you up to some serious health problems. Eating good food needs to be one of the wise choices you make for yourself. Eat foods as close to their natural state as possible. This means fresh fruits and vegetables (organic if possible), whole-grain breads and cereals, less red meat, less fat, more complex carbohydrates, and lots of pure water; go very light on refined sugar, fatty and fried foods, and processed foods. "Junk" food of all kinds can further weaken a body that is already in poor health or lacking in energy.

Helpful hints for giving up worry. Keeping yourself happy by nurturing yourself is the main way to keep from being preoccupied with worry. How to do that is addressed in detail in "Helpful Tips for Getting Out of Burnout" on the facing page. Besides staying happy, there are some other specific things you can do to let worries go.

Ask questions of experienced mothers who have values and a mothering style similar to yours. Then you know that the answers and advice you get will not cause you to worry, and you know that you will not be criticized for your values and parenting style. Surround yourself with supportive friends so you'll have someone with whom you can talk things over. And never spend an entire afternoon worrying over baby when you could call a competent friend for advice.

Remember, you are the best expert on your baby. This means you don't need to read baby magazines to get a lot of advice or another point of view. It's easy to start feeling inadequate and troubled when you expose yourself to material that contradicts what you believe. And remember, baby magazines make their money by being controversial, so many tend to fan the flames of worry rather than put them out! This is especially true for first-time mothers, although I find that I can be vulnerable to this at times even now.

Also, remember, there is no such thing as perfection in parenting. You didn't receive perfect parenting and neither will your children. Every sane parent wants to do the absolute best for his or her child, yet expecting the impossible of yourself is a certain set-up for worry. In this same vein, try not to compare your baby to other babies. As obvious as this sounds, many mothers do it subconsciously, measuring themselves as they see how their baby measures up to their friends' babies. Babies' skills and development will unfold naturally on their own individual timetables. You only make yourself (and your baby!) anxious by wanting him to be smarter, more verbal, more coordinated, and so on.

Avoid things that disturb your peace (partner and child excluded). The TV news is full of local crime or reports of wars overseas. Don't watch it. The world will go on without your knowing about it. (Listen to the radio for the news, if you must, and skip right to the comics in the newspaper if you're having a tough week.) If fashion magazines depress you because you no longer look like you used to, don't read them. If women's magazines and parenting magazines with their "how to do everything better" articles leave you feeling inadequate, don't read them. If the catalogues that arrive in your mail each week are full of things you can't afford, send them unopened into the recycling bin. And if the nice woman you see every day on your morning walk always offers unwanted parenting advice, either change the subject or change your route.

When a crisis develops, ask yourself, "How important is it really?" Ask yourself, "A week from now, or a year from now, or twenty years from now, will it have been worth the worry?" Think of the Alcoholics-Anonymous slogans:

> *One day at a time.*
> *Easy does it.*
> *First things first.*
> *Keep it simple.*
> *Let go and let God.*
> *Live and let live.*

I lost my temper a lot until I learned not to take my child's anger personally and to know when to get help.

● ● ●

As time went on, I realized how important it was for me to maintain a peaceful presence around my child, especially when she was not at peace with herself. What helped was to make a conscious effort to stop complaining and to stop

helpful tips for getting out of burnout

The following is a list of ways to nurture yourself, contributed by many mothers who have experienced periodic burnout and have regained their peace. All have been contributed by mothers who did these activities with their babies. So if your high-need baby can't be left with someone, you still have many creative alternatives for getting your own needs met.

- Take a warm bath.
- Forgive yourself.
- Cook double when you are feeling strong, and freeze one meal.
- Rock in a hammock.
- Get lots of rest.
- Rock in a rocking chair.
- Learn to breast-feed lying down.
- Cook dinner in the morning.
- Swing on a swing.
- Sleep when baby sleeps.
- Limit and coordinate errands.
- Get a foot rub or back rub.
- Even if you can't sleep when the baby sleeps, lie down.
- Run on baby time.
- Get a massage.
- Don't answer the phone.
- Get a haircut.
- Don't watch the clock at night.
- Spend time with good friends.
- Get a manicure or pedicure.
- Take your watch off permanently.
- Eat what you'd eat on holiday.
- Give yourself a facial.
- Treat yourself to an unusual gourmet food or buy some exotic fruit.
- Listen to lullabies.
- Avoid physical overexertion during the day if you know you'll be walking baby around all evening.
- Take time and give yourself permission to just enjoy holding your baby.
- Avoid caffeine.
- Treat yourself to a new purchase – even if it's from a car boot sale or charity shop.
- Seek out people who give you lots of eye contact.
- Set up activities you enjoy at a feeding station (page 149).
- Seek out people who are happy and smile and laugh a lot.
- Write in your baby book.
- Buy a new outfit that's perfect for feeding and lounging.
- Read a mystery.
- Seek out people who support you in your parenting.
- Rent a funny film.
- Learn about mothers in other cultures.
- Read a joke book.
- Avoid people who drain you emotionally.
- Tell jokes.
- Do something you'd do on holiday.
- Play jokes.
- Avoid people who complain a lot.

- Write jokes down so you can remember them.
- Water plants.
- Water the lawn.
- Avoid complaining yourself.
- Enjoy the baby's jokes.
- Concentrate on the present.
- Avoid people who criticize you.
- Start building a library of children's books.
- Take the "shoulds" and "have tos" out of your vocabulary.
- Avoid people who are grumpy and unhappy – even extended family (there will be plenty of time for them later when you're not burned out).
- Listen to upbeat music.
- Do something creative.
- Write letters to friends.
- Don't take on anything that requires a lot of thought.
- Have some fun projects you can easily drop and pick up again to keep you from feeling deprived and to keep you from staring at undone chores.
- Find a support group.
- Get outdoors.
- Pray and enjoy God.
- Take a walk.
- Keep your milk supply up by drinking plenty of fluids.
- Take brisk walks.
- Exercise.
- Limit TV watching.
- With toddlers use water play!
- Dance with your baby.
- Don't watch TV that makes you tense, especially while you're nursing.
- Find a doting four- to six-year-old to keep your toddler company.
- Take a jazzercise or Tumbletots class.
- Enjoy nature.
- Prioritize housework.
- When you and your toddler are ready to leave each other for an hour at a time, spend the time on something you delight in that has nothing to do with mothering.
- Practise relaxation exercises.
- Forget housework.
- Take a shower.
- Set aside periods of time to do nothing (no plans, no commitments) – even fifteen minutes can help.
- Take a bath with baby.
- Avoid or get rid of things that annoy you – bad smells, noisy places.
- Hire a teen.

being exposed to a lot of complaining. I surrounded myself with people who seemed to be in a good mood, and I gently turned the conversation to another topic whenever it was becoming too negative.

Pray or meditate. Being able to connect with your source of spiritual strength and stay peaceful in your spirit is the best antidote for worry. Many women have found motherhood to be a spiritually renewing experience. You may see this as an opportunity for growth on many levels, including spiritual growth and maturity. I have found that God's peace and presence in my life is the one thing I can most fully rely on to keep myself sane and worry-proof. I am a much better mother when I nurture my spiritual foundation. Staying peaceful in the midst of upsetting situations is important not only for my own health, but for the sense of security I want to build in my children. What keeps me motivated is remembering that if my children grow up seeing anxious, worried eyes every day, they grow up believing they are worrisome and anxiety producing.

Helpful hints for nurturing yourself. The items in the box on the previous page comprise an exhaustive (no pun intended) list of ideas. I found a list like this helpful, because often I didn't know what to do to nurture myself. The kind of mother who has the drive to give a lot of nurturing is often a person who is so other-centred she cannot even think of one thing she could do for herself.

Many mothers have found that getting nurturing of the same kind they are giving their babies prevents them from having an empty emotional tank. Ask yourself, "What kind of nurturing am I giving?" A mother of a newborn is holding her baby practically all the time, feeding baby leisurely and often, gazing into baby's eyes, giving lots of affirmation, smiles, encouragement, and empathy. She's helping baby sleep and function well in spite of the discomforts he encounters in life outside the womb. She's rocking, walking, patting, swaying, jiggling, singing lullabies. She spends a lot of time thinking for baby: "You look like you need to be burped, patted, rubbed." So this mother

might need to be held (without pressure for sex) or have a foot rub, a warm bath, or time in a hammock. She needs to have plenty of delicious, nourishing food in the house that she can prepare very easily for herself. She needs to be around encouraging and happy friends who have no expectations of her meeting their needs. She might find it calming to walk outside or listen to soothing music. She'd probably want to avoid tasks that require a lot of thinking, such as planning a week-long camping trip, balancing the chequebook (if it's always messed up), or doing course work for college classes.

The mother of a toddler would have a different set of needs, since she's doing a different type of mothering. She is protecting, encouraging, setting limits, providing alternatives, creating a safe environment for free exploration, saying no a lot, hearing no a lot, comforting, calming, explaining, letting her body be used as a jungle gym, providing nutritious foods, feeding, changing "more interesting" nappies, teaching self-control … So this mother might want to spend some time playing in the sand or in the water, going to a flea market and touching everything, or dancing freely. She'd want to be around encouraging, smiling friends who don't say no and who don't have to be told no. She'd probably want to avoid having to clean up any unnecessary messes that might come from having a puppy or a new pet in the house, or having the lawn dug up.

Give yourself little perks during the day. Rather than have your day revolve around the baby, take him with you to an art museum, a movie, or something YOU like to do.

The idea is to keep filling your emotional tank so it doesn't run dry. Each new day, help yourself have the resources for mothering that you need for that day. You must take responsibility for yourself and your own happiness. It is unwise and unhealthy to give this responsibility to your mate or to your children. A mother who is home all day with her baby can quickly become miserable if she doesn't take charge of herself. One of my friends suggests that a new mother make an agenda for herself each day. She can think of things to do that she enjoys doing and that keep her peaceful. Keep it realistic. Plan to clean out one drawer, write one letter, call a friend, visit a museum, walk in a park. Think about good things. Fill your mind with peaceful thoughts. Resolve to turn negative reflections into positive ones the moment you recognize them.

Knowing your limits is another part of nurturing yourself. This will be especially necessary for the mother of a high-need baby. The extra crying, extra holding, extra nursing, extra everything can easily set you up for some "tear your hair out" time. This may go back to the issue of having to give beyond your personal resources. It is important to recognize when you are being pushed too far so you can take action. Keep it all in perspective.

Helpful hints for dealing with resentment due to unmet expectations. Resentment is a very unhealthy emotion, since it wears you out and accomplishes nothing except setting you up for more resentment. It can get to the point of even causing physical symptoms, like back pains, sore arms, stomachaches, and worse. It becomes part of a vicious cycle, and the only way out of it is to backtrack. Diffuse the source of resentment by discovering just what are the unmet expectations in your life. The next step, of course, is to let go of those expectations. This can be tricky, or downright impossible, without adjusting your attitude toward life in general. Learning to give up worry and to nurture yourself will help with this. Here are some common unmet expectations mothers have had that have caused resentment (the difference between expectation and reality widens with high-need babies):

- I expected my life to be very much the same after the baby was born.
- I expected mothering/breast-feeding to come easily to me.
- I expected to fit the baby into my routine.
- I expected that after six weeks life would be back to normal.
- I expected to be able to do as much housework after the baby was born as before.
- I expected my friends to help/support me after the baby was born.
- I expected it to take less time to feed/care for the baby.
- I expected to be in better shape physically/mentally after the baby was born.
- I expected my partner to help more.
- I expected my baby to sleep more.
- I expected my baby to sleep alone.
- I expected to have more time to myself.
- I expected I would resume a normal sex life sooner.
- I expected to be able to get a shower every day.
- I expected we would all be healthy.

- I expected my baby/toddler to be happy with someone else when I left him.
- I expected my toddler/child would do what I tell her.
- I expected my toddler to potty-train sooner.
- I expected my toddler to eat more.
- I expected my toddler/child would like the foods I prepared for him.
- I expected my baby/toddler/child would play with her toys.
- I expected to resume all my church activities.

You can identify your specific, unmet expectations simply by asking, "What bugs me?" or "What makes me crabby?" Then ask, "Is this a realistic expectation given who I am and what I am doing at this time in my life?" Find out if other mothers have similar frustrations. For example, ask yourself and others, "Is it reasonable, when my baby is five or six months old, to expect to eat my dinner while it's still hot?" Ask other mothers, "If you do it, how do you do it? If you don't, how do you deal with your frustration?" Then ask yourself, "Can I give up this need in my daily routine for a few months or even a few weeks? Is it reasonable to do so? If I can't give up the need, what can I do to anticipate both my need and my baby's need for the next time?" For example: one mother might willingly choose to eat lukewarm food over a ninety-minute mealtime; another will discuss eating in shifts with her partner; another might try eating on the floor while maintaining eye contact with her baby; another will use a music box or toy to distract baby for a few more minutes; another mother might happily learn to eat standing up and swaying to the beat of the Beach Boys.

avoiding mother burnout altogether

Much, if not all, mother burnout can be avoided if you are willing to make some serious changes in the way you manage your day-to-day, minute-by-minute living. These few suggestions are simply what it takes to live a healthy balanced life.

Plan ahead. Anticipation is the key to dealing with many of life's problems, and so it is for avoiding burnout. Plan ahead to nurture yourself. Plan ahead for worries and frustrated expectations by finding a strong support system. Surround yourself with contented, experienced mothers. Have *several* backup plans when things go wrong; for example, if your car is not available on playgroup day, plan another way to get there, or plan to spend that time in another way that keeps you happy. Keep plans simple. Plan rewards for yourself to make up for the inevitable, uncomfortable experiences. Do your planning ahead when you're feeling calm and relatively happy. And remember in your planning to allow twice as much time as before baby to get *anything* done.

Be gentle with yourself. Take the shoulds, how-tos, and musts out of your vocabulary. Replace them with coulds, mights, and maybes. Get up in the morning and connect with your source of peace. Then ask yourself, "What sounds like fun today?" or "What do I feel enthusiastic about?" Then do it. (Remember, keep it simple.) For ideas, look at the box of helpful tips on page 120 and highlight the ones that appeal to you.

Is it selfish to spend so much energy taking care of yourself? Not at all! You are your baby's primary environment. When you care for yourself, you are making an investment in your baby's emotional, physical, and spiritual health.

Your peace of mind helps your family. A baby who feels right within herself becomes a toddler who won't dash away from you, a preschooler who won't be clingy, a school-aged child who is far less likely to be labelled "learning disabled", and a teenager who will not jeopardize his or her future by abusing drugs or having an unwanted pregnancy. When you care for yourself, you are making an investment in your family's well-being, and you set the stage for future generations.

So really be gentle with yourself. Your baby deserves to have a happy mother, not one who is constantly frazzled. Be challenged by the task set before you – to add one healthy, loving child to society – yet keep the challenge from overwhelming you. You can succeed or you would not have been given this child. A burned-out mum can't love herself or her child. You both deserve better.

chapter 8

helping the high-need child go to sleep and stay asleep

High need babies fight sleep; you'll crave sleep. Those are the facts of nighttime parenting with a high-need baby. Sleep, or, more accurately, the lack of it, ranks highest on most parents' complaint lists, and justifiably so. A high-need baby and a seriously under-rested parent are not a healthy match.

Many parents of high-need children have survived the sleepless early months by adopting the attitude, "This sleepless stage won't last forever. I'll simply meet my baby's nighttime needs until he's old enough to meet his own." This outlook is helpful, but it may not be enough. As time goes on, this "nighttime martyr mothering" can easily turn into resentment, which can undermine your whole enjoyment of having a baby. This is why it's necessary to develop creative ways to help your baby sleep at night, just as you work so hard to help him learn to calm himself during the day. (Please notice we didn't say that you expect him to learn this on his own.)

It helps to understand why high-need babies have difficulty sleeping. Most infants, regardless of their need level, have erratic sleeping patterns during the first few months. They have mixed-up days and nights, with frequent feedings and frequent wakings. Yet, as they gradually mature, most infants experience predictable and longer periods of uninterrupted sleep, though each does this at his or her own speed. Studies have shown that babies with easier temperaments go to sleep more easily and stay asleep longer. These babies arrive in the promised land of "Sleep Through the Night" (that is, for at least a five-hour stretch) after a few months. However, high-need babies may not get there for a few years. All babies need their parents at night, and for some, these nighttime needs last longer.

why high-need children sleep differently

"Why do high-need children need more of everything but sleep?" a tired mother once asked me. Until we had a high-need infant, I would have guessed that these babies would be worn out by the end of the day and would actually need more sleep; certainly, their parents do. A tired father once told me, "When it comes to sleep, I'm a high-need parent." Here's why high-need babies sleep differently.

Different temperament. The same tense temperament that causes daytime neediness results in nighttime restlessness. These babies come wired differently, day and night. Their supersensitive nature during the day carries over into their sleep habits during naps and nights. Their keen awareness and curiosity about their environment carries over into being awake and aware at night. It's as though these babies have some internal bright light that stays on all day and isn't easily turned off at night.

From day one, Lauren was incredibly alert. She was not the drowsy newborn I had seen or read about. She would gaze intently at faces, craning her neck to look all around. She was a very light sleeper, too. It was as if she didn't want to waste time sleeping. I would put her down in her infant seat and she would immediately wake up. From the very beginning, she wanted to be either in arms or at the breast constantly, and we obliged her need. We held her during the day, and she slept in my arms at night. I would prop myself up with pillows, and she would sleep in the crook of my arm, lying across my stomach. We slept like this for several weeks, until she got too big for me to be comfortable. I then slowly transitioned her to sleeping beside me on the bed. We slept quite well together. I felt rested during the day and loved having her with us at night.

Different stimulus barrier. Ever wonder why some infants can fall asleep and stay asleep amid the noise of a party, while others awaken when you tiptoe quietly past their bed? This is because babies have different "stimulus barriers", which is the ability to block out disturbing sensory stimuli. Some babies have an amazing ability to block out sensory overload, as if they conclude, "I can't handle all this commotion, I'm tuning out." They fall asleep. High-need babies can't rely on sleep to retreat from sensory overload. Instead, they overreact.

Not only does an immature stimulus barrier keep babies from going to sleep, it interferes with their staying asleep. Infants with a more mature stimulus barrier may sleep through a slight discomfort, such as being too cold, too hot, slightly hungry, or even lonely. These nighttime discomforts awaken high-need babies.

Laurie has always been an extremely light sleeper. I have to unplug the phone, not flush the toilet, not wash dishes, not creak any floors or furniture, not sneeze or cough. Sometimes I feel like I even have to stop breathing as she falls asleep. I can't shift the way I'm holding her or even sit down or stop walking until she is deeply asleep.

Different transitions. High-need babies don't transition easily. They don't willingly switch gears. Going from arms to car seat to arms to shopping trolley is hard for them. Going from the state of being awake to being asleep is a major behavioural transition, one these infants can't make without a lot of help. While you can put some infants down in their cot and they fall asleep, high-need babies have to be deeply asleep before you can put them down. (And when they figure out you put them down when they are deeply asleep, they don't allow themselves to fall deeply asleep anymore.) Even with older high-need children, their minds race so quickly at bedtime (the time *you* assign for them) that they cannot wind down without parental help.

Andrew is now two and a half. He's not breast-feeding anymore, so bedtime has become more of a challenge. For a while, we were able to help him relax with a ritual of bath, stories, and a back rub – off to sleep he went, and I could get up and have some time with Bob. Recently, however, this has changed dramatically. For one thing, Bob is gone some evenings now that he's started his residency. I think Andrew is sensitive to that change. And when Bob is home, he really wants to spend time with me, so I was feeling pressured to get Andrew to sleep. I think Andrew was feeling pressured, too. So it was taking him over an hour to fall asleep, after we'd gone through the bath-and-stories routine. (At least Bob could do that part with him, but Andrew wanted only me to lie down with him.) It seemed he really wasn't ready to go off to sleep, and I wasn't ready to lie there for an hour or more. So I decided to take a more

relaxed approach. We get him all ready for bed (bath and stories) and then Bob and I calmly proceed with our agenda, whether it's just spending time together or reading or watching a programme on TV. Andrew is welcome to be with us; we don't pressure him to stay in the bedroom and go to sleep. We do ask him to spend quiet time, just like we are, and not to disrupt our together time. He feels included in the family circle; and he happily lets me know when he's ready to go to sleep. Or we just take him to bed when we're ready. This is a transition he can handle, no problem. Part of helping him to feel less pressured in transitioning to sleep is leaving the light on in the room until he drops off. We have our light on a dimmer, thank goodness, so it's comfortable for us, too. Thanks, Grandmother Sears, for helping.

Different sleep maturity. Young infants spend much of their sleeping time in a light sleep state, called REM sleep, from which they are easily awakened. During the night infants normally alternate light sleep with deep sleep stages, switching from light sleep to deep sleep and back to light sleep as often as every hour. When making the transition between deep and light sleep, infants go through a vulnerable period in which they are easily awakened. As infants mature, the deep sleep stages lengthen, so that by four to six months, they sleep for longer stretches. High-need babies seem to take longer to develop sleep maturity. They are more prone to awaken during the vulnerable periods of transition from one sleep stage to another. Yet high-need infants often seem to be totally "zonked" when they are in the stage of deep sleep. Eventually, these infants are able to spend more time in deep sleep, yet they do not "sleep through the night" as early as less sensitive babies.

I soon realized that my baby's sleep problem was really society's problem, the fault of its expectations that babies will sleep through the night. My problem was that she wasn't sleeping as expected by me or by the cultural norms.

Different nighttime needs. Craving constant physical contact and not being able to self-soothe are characteristics of high-need babies during the daytime. They are also nighttime features. High-need babies demand whatever daytime and nighttime parenting style gives them a sense of well-being, and that usually means sleeping in physical contact with someone, preferably mother. They won't surrender to any arrangement that takes them out of their mother's arms, not even for a much-needed nap. It seems that they need a womblike environment at night as well as during the day. But just to be inconsistent, as high-need babies get older, the nighttime closeness itself can stimulate them into waking easily while close to mother. High-need babies also have a high degree of separation sensitivity, which can contribute to problems with going to sleep.

He wouldn't settle even sleeping next to me. He had to sleep on me.

don't hurry

Trying to hurry your baby off to sleep is doomed to fail because babies go to sleep differently from adults. In the early months, in order to reach a state of deep sleep, babies need to go through a twenty- to thirty-minute stage of lighter sleep. If you try to put baby down and sneak away during this light sleep stage, he may wake up. You need to continue your ritual until you are certain baby is in a deep sleep. Here's how to tell: watch baby's face and limbs. If baby's mouth is still grimacing or showing "sleep grins", his eyelids are fluttering, and his arms are flexed with hands in fists, baby is still in the state of light sleep. Once baby's face is expressionless, eyes and mouth are still, limbs dangle, and hands are wide open (we call this the "limp-limb sign"), chances are baby has entered deep sleep, and you can put baby down on his back or side and quietly creep away. This is just one of the many facets of baby care that teaches parents patience.

parenting baby to sleep

These different nighttime features of high-need babies do not mean that you must resign yourself to and simply suffer through a year or two of sleeplessness, waiting for your baby to learn to sleep through the night. There are ways you can help your baby, and yourself, get enough sleep.

Teach your child a healthy sleep attitude. High-need infants may fear sleep as a scary time, a time of intense separation anxiety. Teach your infant it's okay to go to sleep, and stay asleep. This means helping your baby develop a healthy sleep attitude: sleep is a pleasant state to enter and a comfortable state to remain in. As much as possible, create a nighttime sleeping environment that is free of night-waking stimuli (physical and emotional). Create a peaceful environment in which to go to sleep, *conditioning* baby to sleep under the conditions that help him relax into sleep. Remember, sleep is not a state you can force your baby into. It must naturally overtake baby.

Helping your baby develop a healthy sleep attitude means also developing one of your own. Certainly, it's normal to wish for an uninterrupted night's sleep, it's normal to resent your baby's night waking, and it's normal to long for a time of being free of a baby who clings all day long. Try not to let these feelings override your long-term goal: a child who grows up with healthy sleep habits. Otherwise, in desperation to get some much-needed sleep, you may fall prey to the quick-fix methods of "sleep training" that are likely to create a distance between you and your baby, and also place your baby at risk for developing an unhealthy sleep attitude. Besides, high-need babies are notoriously resistant to quick fixes and sleep-training methods that rely on gadgets and crying it out. (See related section "Should Baby Cry It Out?" pages 37–8.) Letting yourself be lured into quick-fix sleep-training methods keeps you from continuing to work at finding sleeping arrangements and a nighttime parenting style that meet everyone's nighttime needs. Good sleepers are partly born, partly made, but never forced to give up and go to sleep. Enter nighttime parenting with an open mind toward working at whatever arrangement gets all of you a good night's sleep. And keep working at it. What does not work at one stage may work at another. There is no right or wrong sleeping arrangement for every baby – only the right ones for your family.

Consider medical causes of night waking. If your infant awakens in pain (sudden shrieks, inconsolable crying) and is not easily resettled by your usual comforting measures, suspect your baby is hurting (see Chapter 10, "Hidden Causes of Fussiness in Infants"). In our paediatric practice, we have seen hundreds of infants who were unfairly diagnosed with "night-waking problems" and were prescribed the unhelpful cry-it-out advice. After investigating these babies for medical causes of nighttime pain and prescribing a more appropriate treatment, these infants slept better.

Mellow baby during the day. We have noticed a correlation between how much holding, rocking, and gentling babies receive during the day and how well they sleep at night. The baby who is worn in a sling close to a parent several hours a day and has a lot of skin-to-skin contact during feeding is likely to reward his parents' daytime investment with a less wakeful night.

Arrive at a sleeping arrangement that works.*
Where should baby sleep, in a cot in his own room, in a cot in your room, or with you in your bed? Answer: baby should sleep wherever the whole family sleeps best. Experiment with various sleeping arrangements until you find one that works for everyone. And keep your options open. Where you and your baby get the most restful night's sleep may change from month to month as your baby's nighttime needs change and sleep patterns mature.

Having tried both putting our baby in her cot and sleeping with her in our bed, I can definitely say that the latter is for me. It's the only way to care for our fussy, sensitive, wakeful baby. It did, however, take us a couple of months to adjust our lifestyle to the routine involved in having our baby sleep with us. Even now I have to go to bed at about the same time she does to feel well rested. In addition to getting enough rest and meeting her needs, the big advantage to sleeping with my baby is I have learned to go to sleep much more quickly and sleep more efficiently. I really enjoy having Alex cuddled next to me at night. I'm so glad I didn't miss out on this special closeness with her.

Parent your baby to sleep. Notice we said, "parent", not just "put", your baby to sleep. If you expect to put an awake baby down into a cot, say "night-night", and walk out of the room, forget it. This is an unrealistic expectation for most babies, and it rarely (if ever) is the sleep profile of

a high-need baby. As we mentioned on page 128, high-need babies don't transition easily from being awake to being asleep. Most will need to go to sleep in arms, at the breast, in the car, in the sling, or on the shoulder of a parent. The key to parenting your baby to sleep is to develop a repertoire of sleep-inducing rituals that help baby relax into sleep and give baby the message "It's time to go to sleep." Sleep rituals capitalize on a principle called a "setting event", in which the first scene of the ritual leads baby to expect the whole series of pleasant interactions that ultimately lead to sleep. Since with high-need infants what worked one month might not work the next, be willing to change your ritual. Here are the top sleep-inducers that have worked in our family or in families from our paediatric practice.

Massaging and bathing. Infant massage on a towel, on your lap, or on the floor in a warm place before or after a warm bath is a wonderful ritual to relax tense muscles and unwind busy minds. See the related section "Infant Massage", page 73.

Nursing down. "Nursing" implies soothing an infant, whether by breast or bottle. Drifting off to sleep at mother's breast is a proven sleep-inducing winner. Nurse your baby in a rocking chair or lying next to him on your bed. Baby has already learned to associate breast-feeding with calming. Your milk contains natural sleep inducers, and the hormones stimulated by the act of breast-feeding also relax you.

Drifting off to sleep in warm arms, sucking from a bottle of warm formula, hearing a warm

---

* The advantages and practical how-to suggestions on sleeping with your baby are fully discussed in *The Baby Book*, by William Sears and Martha Sears (Thorsons 2005).

lullaby while moving back and forth in a rocking chair will also help sleep overtake the unwilling baby in a beautiful, gentle way.

Whether you are breast- or bottle-feeding, be aware that if your arms are tense, baby will pick up your tension. Use a pillow under the arm holding baby so you can relax your muscles.

Once I changed my attitude about getting up at night, our relationship improved. Instead of resenting this intrusion into my sleep, I realized what a special, uninterrupted bonding time it was to sit in a rocking chair and just nurse and caress her with no one to interrupt. I realized that these were precious moments that I may never again have. For us, this was really quality time.

Slinging down. This sleep-inducing technique was a lifesaver for winding down Sears infants who were not quite ready to go to sleep, even though we were ready to put them down. When you feel baby is ready for bed (though baby may not agree), cradle or snuggle her in a sling. (The forward-facing position can be too stimulating to send a baby off to sleep, yet some high-need babies won't accept any other position; it's as if they know they're going to fall asleep if they are all snuggled up.) Stroll around quietly until baby falls asleep. (This will take longer if baby is facing forward.) If necessary, you can get some household tasks done during this ritual. If baby doesn't relax because he "knows what's up", go for a walk outside. Ten minutes outside in the sling is usually worth forty-five minutes of trying to rock baby to sleep in the rocking chair. As soon as you feel confident that baby is in a deep sleep (see limp-limb sign, described in the

"Don't Hurry" box on page 129), walk slowly to the bed, bend over, and ease yourself out of the sling while lowering the baby onto the mattress. Snuggle the sling around the baby to ease the transition. Wearing baby down in a sling is a useful way to help a baby through the transition from being hyper-stimulated and awake to being in a state of deep sleep. Sometimes when you think baby is in a deep sleep, he will awaken as soon as you put him down. He may need to continue physical contact with you for a while longer. In that case, keep baby in the sling and lie down with him, letting him drape across your chest or snuggle next to you. The rhythm of your breathing and heartbeat will allow sleep to completely overtake baby. Then, roll over carefully while slipping yourself out of the sling and quietly ease away – if you haven't drifted off to sleep yourself.

Mutual napping. Wearing down is particularly useful for the reluctant napper. When baby falls asleep in the sling, snuggled with his tummy against your chest or draped over your chest once you lie down, you both can take a much-needed mutual nap.

All of the above. Many smart high-need babies hold out for all of the above (and more) nighttime parenting techniques. Put yourself in the place of a busy baby not wanting to give up the play delights of the day or the physical attractions of being in the arms and at the breasts of the person she loves. This baby likes to be soothed by a warm bath and a relaxing massage followed by a walk in the sling. She may want to nurse while riding in the sling, and then nurse some more lying down. Going from a warm bath to warm arms to warm breasts to a warm bed is a wonderful way for babies to go to sleep. What better routine for building a healthy sleep attitude and storing away pleasant nighttime memories?

Fathering down. In order to thrive and survive with a high-need baby, both parents must share the daytime and the nighttime parenting. Even the most experienced mothers often fall into the solo nighttime-parenting trap, for several reasons. First, mothers feel they can soothe their baby off to sleep and put him back to sleep more quickly and easily than father can, and usually this is the case. Second, breast-feeding mothers have a monopoly on the most useful sleep-inducing tool, the breast. Third, mothers take pity on their partners, placing a high priority on dad's need for an uninterrupted night's sleep so that he can function well on the job the next day. (However, mothers also need a restful night's sleep to function at their job the next day, whether it be in or outside the home.) Fourth, new fathers have a remarkable capability for becoming deaf after midnight. Some dads can actually sleep through even the most ear-piercing cries, while mothers usually awaken at the first whimper.

There was a time when Lon was in charge of Kris (age four) at night, and I was in charge of baby Eliza. Lon could sleep through Eliza's crying (and she was really loud), but would wake for a tiny noise from Kris in another room, which I usually slept through.

Differences in nighttime hearing ability don't let fathers off the hook. Some babies, though not many high-need babies, can get used to the parenting-to-bed rituals of both mum and dad. One is usually not better than the other, they're just different, and babies can learn different approaches. If baby resists dad's ministrations, don't despair. Baby will get used to dad and other ways of going to sleep when it's developmentally appropriate, between eighteen months and two-and-a-half to three years. If there comes a time when you absolutely have to get a catch-up night's sleep, it may be very difficult for dad to take over. But you'll be surprised what unique ways of comforting babies men can come up with when they have to. Necessity is the mother (and father) of invention. (See related sections "The Warm Fuzzy", and "The Neck Nestle", page 74.)

Swinging down. Wind-up swings for winding down babies are a boon to parents who have neither the time and energy nor creativity to muster up rituals of their own. Tired parents will pay anything for a good night's sleep. Once in a while a moving plastic seat may be more sleep-inducing than a familiar pair of arms. Sometimes high-need babies associate a parent's body with play and stimulation and will not drift off to sleep in a human swing. For them the mechanical one is less stimulating, if not downright boring, and therefore can be a useful part of a sleep-ritual repertoire. Yet remember, high-need babies are notoriously resistant to mechanical mother substitutes and will usually protest anything less than the real mum. Before you actually spend money on a swing, you might want to borrow one for a week or two to see if the spell of the swing will last. You may discover that you are uncomfortable with mechanical mothering and decide to get more creative. Still, swings have their moments.

Nestling down. If you've tried all of the above suggestions and your baby still won't settle, it may be that your baby is just not ready to go to sleep or is ready but does not want to sleep alone. If you really need to get to sleep yourself, you may have to create an environment of super-womb: lie down next to your baby, snuggle up face-to-face (or face-to-breast), and drift off to sleep with your baby in your arms and/or feeding at your breast. If the arm under baby gets cramped or full of pins and needles, move it over your head and cuddle your baby with your top arm. Put a pillow behind your lower back for support. This is a warm and reassuring way for baby to go off to sleep, yet it also creates a no-nonsense environment in which sleep will overtake the reluctant baby. I have many beautiful memories of Martha and our babies going to sleep this way. As I stood at the bedside observing the sleeping pair, I couldn't help thinking, "Now, there's a smart baby."

Wheeling down (or driving down). Suppose you've exhausted all of the above human-contact ways of getting your baby to sleep, yet you know your baby needs to go to sleep (or at least you need your baby to go to sleep). Start the car. Put your baby in a car seat and drive non-stop for as long as it takes to get your baby to sleep, usually at least twenty minutes. We call

this before-bed ritual "motorway fathering" (see page 64). This method of getting baby to sleep has been a long time winner in the Sears family. Our oldest son, Jim, once had a summer job typing the manuscript for a series of articles I was writing on fathering, one of which included a discussion of motorway fathering. This method stuck in Jim's mind, and he tried it out ten years later when he became a father. I was flattered.

keeping baby asleep

High-need babies need help not only falling asleep but often staying asleep. Here are ways to keep them asleep so that you can stay asleep, too.

Sleep where baby sleeps best. As we discussed on page 131, every mum, dad, and baby must work out and keep evaluating the sleeping arrangement that gets everyone a restful night's sleep most of the time. Some high-need babies seem to have a critical distance for contented sleeping. For some, sleeping too far away from their parents gives them an acute case of nighttime separation anxiety, causing them to awaken frequently. Other babies seem to get stimulated by sleeping too close to their parents, and awaken frequently there. (Of course, some parents may not realize how much a normal breast-fed baby wakes up.) Parents also vary in the amount of nighttime attachment that gives them the most restful night's sleep. Some mothers do not sleep well with their babies too

nighttime spoiling?

A modern theory about babies' sleep problems is that if a baby relies on the presence of the parent to go to sleep, he will never learn to go to sleep on his own, and he will expect the same person to be there to put him back to sleep if he wakes up in the middle of the night. Thus, baby will never learn to settle himself back to sleep either. This belief is related to the old "spoiling" theory, but it is also based on the concept of "sleep associations" – people, things, and activities adults use to help themselves relax and sleep. Adults have favourite sleep associations – a familiar bed with comfy sheets and their favourite pillow, a book, music, and so on; but most adults are able to go back to sleep in the middle of the night without repeating the associations they used to get to sleep (unless, perhaps, the comfy pillow or familiar bed is not there, as in a hotel). Babies, however, often can't resettle on their own; they rely on people or props to get them back to sleep. The sleep-association concept accounts for mothers and fathers fearing nighttime dependency ("I don't want him to get into the habit of always sleeping in our bed or of my feeding him to sleep"). I once saw a mother whose baby was sleeping quite well, as long as the infant fed down to sleep and slept nestled next to mother. Parents and baby were both sleeping fine, and this attachment relationship was working for them. I advised the parents to continue this beautiful relationship and said they would see healthy benefits later on. However, the fear of future nighttime dependency led these parents to seek a second opinion from a "sleep specialist", who diagnosed a "sleep-association disorder". It never dawned on me to consider a human, high-touch nighttime family snuggle as a disorder, but that's what happens when adult standards are mistakenly applied to tiny babies.

As the father of eight children, most of whom shared our bed for several years, I can assure parents that offspring do eventually learn to sleep without parents' presence. The pleasant sleep associations they learn from sharing sleep minimize sleep problems later on. They don't fight sleep, they welcome it.

far away from them, some fathers do not sleep well with their infants too close, and sometimes both parents are very anxious about one extreme or the other.

When baby sleeps too close to me, he fusses. When he sleeps too far from me, he fusses. I keep

experimenting with different sleeping distances, and it changes from week to week.

• • •

There came a point when exhaustion overwhelmed me. Our other two children had slept with us as babies, but I was afraid to put our three-pound, thirteen-ounce premature baby in bed with me. I feared I'd fall asleep and my breast would smother her. Her nose was the size of the tip of my pinkie. But one night after weeks of walking the floor with a crying baby, I snuggled her in bed with me and figured one night without the "preemie routine" of breast pumping and supplemental bottles would be okay. We were there for seven hours. It was heaven! From then on, we went to bed together, and we slept! She would nurse frequently during the night, but she never cried. This was the beginning of our sharing sleep together. I was amazed at her need for physical closeness to me, despite the fact that she'd spent most of her short life alone in ICU. I embraced this need with joy. Those primal instincts are not easily squelched. I began to see her high-need personality as a positive sign; looking on the bright side, high-need babies have finely tuned survival instincts.

● ● ●

I resisted any idea of sleeping with my baby until one night I thought, well, we slept together for nine months and it didn't kill either of us. Defying everything I had been told, and following my instincts, I took her to bed with me – and we slept!

Vary your nighttime response. Whether night waking is the result of a need or a habit is a judgment call, and a difficult one. Babies would claim they need comfort; sleep trainers claim it's a habit. The goal of nighttime parenting is to make it more attractive for baby to stay asleep than to wake up.

For example, if your toddler awakens and you "reward" the awakening, you set yourself up for many more wakeful nights. Yet it's a natural maternal instinct, especially for a breast-feeding first-time mother, to rush to comfort a toddler back to sleep using his favourite pacifier. Suppose each time you awakened, your favourite person instantly rewarded you with your favourite treat. How motivated would you be to stay asleep?

At the other extreme is playing deaf to all night waking, to let baby "cry it out" and "break the night-waking habit". This is common advice given by sleep trainers and well-meaning friends who are not there at 3am and who have no connection to the baby who is awakening. Few mothers are able to be insensitive to their baby's nighttime needs, and besides, most high-need babies will outlast any scheme to let them cry it out. They just keep on crying. They don't learn to put themselves back to sleep. They just get angry and frightened.

It helps to have a variety of ways to comfort night wakers, so baby will learn that nighttime needs can be met in many different ways. Develop a large repertoire of nighttime responses depending on the age of your baby:

- feeding (a newborn needs to be fed; a one-year-old probably doesn't)
- sucking
- tummy-patting
- singing a lullaby
- rocking
- snuggling
- reassuring voices

For nighttime sanity's sake, it's helpful for mother and father to share nighttime comforting. You'll appreciate one another rather than resent one another.

We took shifts during the nighttime hours. I would get up and nurse her or I'd just pull her next to me in bed. If she wouldn't fall asleep, Michael would walk with her or we would just both get up together. Sometimes we'd watch a hilarious 3am. television show. If Michael was walking with her, then I'd get some letters written or do some reading, and make it productive time instead of just feeling frustrated that it was a waste.

Realistically, high-need babies are notoriously resistant to most nighttime tricks, especially the popular sleep-training strategies, which are just modern versions of the same old cry-it-out method. Remember, these babies have a strong mind-set. They want what they want, and any alternative is met with a wailing protest. If babies awaken expecting their mother's breasts but get a plastic plug instead, most high-need babies will indignantly protest your trick to the entire neighbourhood.

Keep in mind that your goal is to condition your child to sleep, not awaken. Try to meet his nighttime needs in a relaxed and boring fashion. Give him a sense that nighttime is different from day and that we don't play in the middle of the night. It's not that you don't meet your baby's needs at night, but you recognize that the main need at this time is for sleep and a well-rested mother in the morning. Once again, what helps to keep you calm so you can truly help baby be calm is to let go of the expectation that you should be getting an uninterrupted eight-hour stretch of sleep.

I feel that in our society we lose more sleep over the battle we set up, and the anger that ensues, than the actual time it takes to parent a baby back to sleep.

Time your response and be boring. Keep working at your cry response until you find the one that resettles your baby the fastest and disturbs your rest the least. Some mothers find a *quick response* works best; they know from experience that those first sounds will escalate into a family-arousing wail if ignored. At the first whimper, you immediately comfort your baby by letting him suck, patting his tummy, holding him, rocking him, singing softly to him, placing your hand on his tummy, which puts pressure on him to make him feel held and warm, rocking the cradle – whatever works *before* baby (and you) completely awaken. If baby is in bed next to you, try hugging him in close to you in the teddy bear snuggle (see page 75). Bottle-fed babies may settle if you help them find a thumb or dummy. Sometimes just helping an older baby find a better sleep position works. This quick-response approach works best if baby is nearby or in your bed rather than in his own room, unless you have a very sensitive monitor and sleep with one ear awake.

Other mothers find the *slow response* works better. If you don't rush in to comfort baby at the first whimper, baby may not awaken fully and will drift back into deep sleep without intervention or may awaken and resettle herself back to sleep without your help. Babies with easier temperaments and older babies are more likely to resettle themselves.

There are risks and benefits to both approaches. Responding too quickly may reward an older baby for waking and short-circuit his developing ability to self-comfort. Responding too slowly allows baby to fully awaken and become frightened or angry at your slow response. This will make it more difficult to settle baby and yourself back to sleep. Somewhere between these extremes is the right response for your family, and it may change at each stage of baby's development.

When comforting a night-waker, try not to reinforce the waking. If you rush in with a panicky voice and scoop up baby in tense arms, you convey that there really is something to be scared about at night. Instead, be quiet, calm, soothing while you give an "It's OK to sleep" message.

Detect irritants that could cause restlessness.
Remember, many high-need babies are hypersensitive to noise and uncomfortable irritants. While most infants are not awakened by these stimuli, supersensitive babies are. As much as you can, minimize noises that startle, and bodily discomforts that irritate. This requires putting on your detective cap, analysing your baby's sleeping environment, and, as much as possible, removing any stimuli that could awaken baby. Use the following checklist as your guide.

- **Stuffy noses.** Plugged noses awaken tiny babies. Babies under six months don't readily switch to mouth-breathing if their noses are plugged. Keep baby's sleeping environment as free of nasal irritants as possible (cigarette smoke, animal dander, perfumes or hairspray, mould, mildew, chemical odours, dust from stuffed animals, etc.). Clues that a nighttime stuffy nose is the problem include persistent restlessness; noisy, throaty breathing; and difficulty feeding at night. In addition to removing possible nasal irritants, "hose your baby's nose" before bedtime, using over-the-counter saltwater nose drops and an infant nasal-suction bulb.
- **Irritating sleepwear.** Some babies cannot settle in synthetic sleepwear. Change to 100 per cent cotton clothing to see if your baby sleeps better.
- **Environmental irritants.** The same things that can cause a stuffy nose (see above) can also cause a general irritability at night. If you've ever experienced a tickle far back on your palate that you can't get to, you'll have some idea what an internal irritation can do to disturb baby's sleep. This irritation may be present at other times besides sleep time, but baby won't usually notice it in his busy waking hours. Like teething pains, physical discomfort is so much worse at night because there is no distraction from it.
- **Dietary sensitivities.** Hypersensitive babies may have food intolerances. See Chapter 10 for help detecting which foods may be disturbing baby's delicate system. Like environmental irritants, certain foods in baby's diet (and your diet while you are breast-feeding) can cause internal irritation.
- **Night pains.** Consider the physical cause of restlessness described in Chapter 10.
- **Startling noises.** Sounds that are sudden, loud, and *unfamiliar* awaken supersensitive babies. Oil squeaky cots; warn older siblings not to slam doors; remove noisy clocks; and so on. For sounds that may settle them, see pages 70–1.

I wish to thank you for your sensitivity and intuition as Ian's doctor. When I brought him in to see you, I was beside myself, at the end of my rope. He hardly slept at all during the day or at night. At night it was the worst. From 8:00pm till 2:00am, he would tense up, pull his knees up to his chest, and scream. It was impossible to calm him, hold him, or even feed him. I tried everything – swinging, rocking, walking, and sleeping with him. The list is endless. I refused to believe he was colicky. I explained to you what he did, and you said it sounded like something external rather than internal.

I realized that the only time he was content was when we changed him and he had no clothes on. I was putting him in 100 per cent polyester nightwear in the evenings, and that was when he was the worst. He was totally miserable. During the day he was usually in something 50/50 cotton/polyester, and he was less miserable.

So I went home and put him in 100 per cent cotton nappies, clothes, blanket, and bedding. I couldn't believe it! I had a new baby in my arms. He was totally calm and content. He even started cooing and smiling and seemed happy. I thought it was too good to be true, but the next day he even took several naps! Just like a real baby!

He is finally out of his misery. I am so glad we didn't just write him off as a colicky baby. I can now enjoy my baby. He is now a happy, content, cooing, and smiling baby!

• • •

When our first baby woke up wet during the night, I would take her into the changing room, turn the lights on, take off her wet nappy, clean her, and put a new nappy on. By that time, she was totally awake and I had to feed her back to sleep. With our second baby, a friend of mine convinced me I didn't have to change a baby's nappy during the night. Initially, I was afraid it would leak all over the place and the whole bed would get wet, but here's what I did. I covered her bottom with a zinc oxide barrier cream, put three cloth nappies on her, and sometimes even used a nappy cover. When she woke up at night I didn't change her. I just pulled her next to me and fed her. I did everything I could to keep it quiet and dark and un-stimulating.

• • •

I wrapped Philip in a nice warm blanket so that only his head poked out right before I fed him to sleep in the rocking chair. That way, when I went to put him down, he still felt warm and secure. I took that a step further and put flannel sheets on our king-size bed so that the sheets wouldn't be so cold as to wake him up when I put him down.

Nurse throughout the night. In my practice, some mothers relate that their high-need babies and toddlers seem to feed a lot at night. How you approach this depends on how old the baby is and whether or not you are actually waking up feeling sufficiently rested (remember "motherzone", page 19). First refer to Chapter 10, "Hidden Causes of Fussiness in Infants". A baby of any age deserves to have his night waking investigated for medical and physical causes. Younger babies almost always have concrete problems (even to our adult minds) that cause waking, such as hunger, and they sleep much better once these problems are addressed.

We found in our own experience with high-need babies that as they became toddlers, the amount of night waking Martha was able to handle changed. When Erin was a bit past two, Martha began setting limits on night nursing because she was pregnant and needed her sleep. She literally could not stand lengthy feedings, especially at night, so she'd let Erin nurse for two or three minutes and then ask her to stop (Erin was not always willing), and Martha cuddled her up close. What saved the situation was that Martha discovered that Erin would relax if she could put her hand on Martha's breast. In fact, she fell asleep faster doing this than if she was allowed to keep sucking. Martha also discovered that Erin relaxed and went off to sleep much more quickly when Martha was able to stay peaceful herself.

When Matthew hit this stage, Martha was not pregnant again yet, but still felt desperate for sleep if awakened more than two or three times. I would wake up to hear a dialogue like "Nee" (his word for nurse) … "No" … "Nee!" … "No!" … "Nee!!" … "No, not now. In the morning. Mummy's sleeping. You sleep, too." A firm but calm, peaceful voice almost always did the trick. You can manage to stay peaceful in this situation when you know you are not damaging your very secure, attachment-parented child, and you also know what will happen if you don't stay peaceful.

When Stephen was around twenty months, he was typically nursing twice at night, occasionally three times, and Martha was fine with this. Actually, she found it enjoyable. But he hit a stage when he started waking four and five times, and Martha tried the calm, peaceful "No" dialogue. Every child is different, and Stephen wasn't buying it. So we devised the plan we wrote about in *The Baby Book*. Martha would nurse Stephen the first two times he woke. Then if it was still a long time till morning, I would pick him up and walk with him the next time. He cried, but it did not escalate to panic, and I lasted him out. After nearly an hour he fell back to sleep in my arms and I laid him back down next to a sleeping Martha. After three or four nights (with less and less crying each night), he stopped the frequent waking, and all was well again. And stayed well. He learned what our limits were!

In some families with different temperaments and levels of ability to cope, we have learned that this "cry-it-out-in-dad's-arms" advice may not work. One mum had this to say:

Not every toddler waking frequently at night to nurse will do well crying it out in dad's arms. What he may need is to learn to sleep alone on a separate mattress or with a sibling, because the proximity to mum is stimulating the waking. It's time for a positive weaning from the family bed, not a negative "you're-stuck-with-dad" experience.

We have learned that the "just say no" approach also isn't right for all toddlers. I was on a talk show once giving this suggestion to a caller who had a sixteen-month-old waking two to five times a night. A week later I got a letter from a mother who had identified with this caller's situation and had tried out the advice herself. She was amazed at how well it seemed to be working and wrote to thank me. However, a few weeks later she called Martha, very confused because everything had deteriorated. Her sixteen-month-old, who had actually managed to sleep for nine hours with one or two brief wakings of a few seconds without breast-feeding, was now a very clingy, weepy child by day. She wondered if it was connected to the night situation. Martha helped her understand that during a weaning of any kind, it is important to look at the overall effect on the child. Any drastic change in nighttime routine needs to be assessed by how it affects the child's daytime behaviour. She included the insight that radio talk shows cannot allow for a complete exploration of problems and solutions (especially when the adviser is male and the show's host is male!). Her next thank-you letter (addressed to Martha this time) said, "You really helped me put it all into perspective! I've become a much more 'go with the flow' and intuitive parent. Not letting my daughter breast-feed at all during the night was clearly too much for her to handle right now." In my defence, I didn't mean to imply that the other mother not nurse her baby *at all* at night, but I guess that's what came across.

Our youngest child, Lauren, is ours by adoption. Though she breast-fed for nine months, she didn't wake to nurse during the night after the first few months. Thankfully, she was usually a "good sleeper"; yet there were times when she would wake and think it was time to play, or times that she was sick and

couldn't get back to sleep. The old standby of offering a breast was not an option. Martha, by now an expert on not having nighttime expectations, would simply get up with her and take her down to the living room, where no one else would be disturbed. She'd rock Lauren or let her play in the dark while Martha would lie on the couch and rest.

alternatives for the all-night nurser

Frequent night nursing is the most common situation that brings parents of high-need toddlers to our surgery for counselling.

Remember, it's the nature of high-need children to demand whatever they believe they need for their well-being. Frequent night nursing is characteristic of high-need children. It's like going to their favourite restaurant. The ambiance is peaceful, the server is familiar, the cuisine is superb, and they love the management. Who can blame the all-night gourmet? Try these suggestions for dealing with all-night nursing:

Assess the situation. How much of a problem is the frequent night nursing? This stage of high-level night nurturing will pass. Both you and your baby will someday sleep through the night. Yet if you are sleep-deprived to the degree that you are barely functioning the next day, you resent your nighttime parenting style (and your baby), and the rest of your family relationships are deteriorating, you need to make some changes in your nighttime feeding schedule. Even if you can't get your baby to sleep through the whole night, you can help him cut back on nighttime nursing, making the situation more tolerable for you. Here's how:

Tank your baby up during the day. Toddlers love to breast-feed, yet they are often so busy during the day that they forget to feed. Or mum is so busy that she forgets to feed. But at night, there you are, only an inch away, and baby wants to make up for missed daytime feedings. (This is a common scenario when a breast-feeding mother returns to work outside the home.) Finding more time to feed during the day may make the breast less attractive at night.

Increase daytime touch. Wear your baby in a sling and give your baby more touch time during the day. (See suggestions for baby-wearing, pages 55–6.) It's easy when babies get older to greatly decrease the amount of touching time without realizing it. All-night feeding can sometimes be a baby's signal reminding mothers not to rush their baby into independence. In developing a healthy independence, a child goes out and comes back, lets go and clings, step by step until she is going out more than she is coming back. Many mothers have noted that babies and toddlers show an increased need for feeding or holding right before undertaking a new stage of development, such as crawling, walking, staying with a sitter, and so on.

Awaken baby for a full feed just before you go to bed. Rather than going off to sleep only to be wakened an hour or two later, get in a feed just as you begin your time in bed. This way, your sleep will be disturbed one fewer times, and you'll (hopefully) have a longer stretch of sleep to begin your night. This doesn't work if you don't have a full feeding to give at this time, so be certain to keep your milk supply up. Call your local breast-feeding counsellor for tips.

"Nummies go night-night." Now the marketing begins. Around eighteen months, your child has the capacity to understand simple sentences. Programme your toddler not to expect to be nursed when she awakens, such as by saying, "We'll nurse again when Mr Sun comes up." When you nurse her to sleep (or have the first or second night nursing), the last thing she should hear is "Mummy go night-night, Daddy go night-night, baby go night-night, and nummies go night-night" (or whatever are her favourite comforters). When she wakes during the night, the first thing she should hear is a gentle reminder, "Nummies are night-night. Baby go night-night, too." This programme may require a week or two of repetition. Soon she will get the message that daytime is for feeding and nighttime is for sleeping. If "nummies" stay night-night, baby will too – at least till dawn.

Remember, toddlers are searching for a norm. They want to know what standard of behaviour is expected in their home. It's up to you to teach them the norm. If night nursing is the norm, they will continue to expect and enjoy this delightful nighttime interaction. If they learn that mum's café closes at bedtime, they will come to accept this as the norm.

Offer a substitute. High-need babies are not easily fooled; they don't readily accept substitutes. Yet, sometimes it's worth trying. Remember, nursing does not always mean breast-feeding. Honour your partner with his share of "night nursing", so your toddler does not always expect to be comforted by nummies. This gives dad a chance to develop creative nighttime fathering skills, and the child a chance to expand her acceptance of nighttime comforters. To enable baby to accept dad's nighttime comforting, mother may need to sleep in another room for a couple of nights.

Increase the sleeping distance between you. If the above suggestions do not entice your persistent night nurser to cut back, yet you still feel you must encourage him to do so, try another sleeping arrangement, such as putting him on a mattress or futon at the foot of your bed, or even having him sleep in another room, perhaps with a sibling. Dad or mum can lie down beside baby to comfort him if he awakens. Mum can even nurse, if necessary, but sneak back to her own bed if continued closeness seems to encourage continued waking.

Let baby be the barometer. When trying any behaviour-changing technique on a child, don't persist with a bad experiment. Use your baby's daytime behaviour as a barometer of whether your change in nighttime parenting style is working. If after several nights of working on night weaning your baby is her same self during the day, then persist with your gradual night weaning. If, however, she becomes more clingy, whiny, or distant, take this as a clue to slow down your rate of night weaning. Here's where your previous training in baby reading will really pay off.

Babies will wean, and someday they will sleep through the night. This high-maintenance stage of nighttime parenting will pass. The time in your arms, at your breast, and in your bed is a relatively short while in your child's whole life (and yours!), yet the memories of love and availability last forever.

chapter 9

feeding high-need children

In counselling hundreds of parents of high-need babies we have been impressed with the feeding challenges these infants present. It seems that the overall super-sensitivity of these infants carries over into sensitivity to foods and feeding techniques. Feeding infants, especially high-need ones, is not only a nutritional necessity, it's a social interaction.

You will spend more time feeding your infant than in any other single interaction – except comforting. Here's how to enjoy those special feeding times.

the benefits of breast-feeding

Breast-fed babies fuss less than bottle-fed, and breast-feeding mothers are more able to cope with their baby's high needs. Here's why:

Baby receives more touch. Being held and enjoying skin contact are lifesavers for these infants. Because breast milk is digested more rapidly than formula, breast-fed babies are fed more often, so they get held more. A breast-feeding mother is more likely to respond quickly to her baby's distress. She offers the breast as a source of comfort, almost by reflex without the mental exercise of deciding what to do. Bottle-feeding mothers are more likely to think in terms of specific feeding times and employ alternative ways of comforting the baby between feedings (many of which tend to require putting baby down). High-need babies soon learn to use the breast as a readily available and lovingly offered source of comfort. Nearly every mother of a high-need baby volunteers, "My baby wants to feed all the time." Can you blame these smart little infants? What a nice, soft, warm place to snuggle! What sweet, fresh milk!

Because of criticism and advice, I made a very big mistake when Julia was nine months old. Friends encouraged me to quit breast-feeding because they "knew" that the source of her crying and frustration was hunger. These more "experienced" mums said that my breast milk was not sufficient for her appetite. I conceded and weaned her, and waited for things to get better. They got worse. Then, after weaning her, I realized that breast-feeding was one of the few tools that both Julia and I had had available to calm her. It was about the only thing that had worked, regardless of how attached that kept us. Now it was a tool I no longer had at my disposal. And I can't tell you how much anguish and frustration I tolerated through the weaning process in hopes of a solution. Score: friends, one – me, zero. Moral: Don't stop breast-feeding! Don't listen to others. Listen to your heart.

Baby experiences fewer allergies and intestinal discomforts. Formula intolerance is a frequent cause of infant discomfort. Infants react to the cow's milk or soy protein in formulas. Formula-fed infants are more prone to constipation, seldom a problem with breast-fed babies. (See the related discussion of food and milk sensitivities in Chapter 10.)

Mother's sensitivity increases. During those marathon days when baby wants to feed all day and night, it's normal for you to feel that you are giving, giving, giving, and all "gived out". Yet, by frequent feeding, baby also gives something to you. Breast-feeding gives you the extra boost of maternal hormones that increase your sensitivity to your baby. Breast-feeding also helps you become more intuitive. It is an exercise in baby reading that is repeated frequently throughout the day. You must learn to read your baby's cues and trust her ability to communicate if you are going to succeed at breast-feeding. And that ability to read your child will serve you well in the years to come.

We're in harmony with each other. I nurse an average of twelve times a day. I know this sounds like a lot of nursing, but there is never a schedule to it. Either she lets me know or I just start it. It always works out. Nursing is never a hassle or bother. It's just second nature to me. Breast-feeding is my salvation because it is most often the comforting tool that works, and I don't know what I would do without it. It's so rewarding to see her content while she is nursing. It also relaxes me, and helps us connect. It helps me feel in tune with her. Breast-feeding forces me, a compulsive cleaner, to sit with her whenever she wants to nurse. It assures her that the same person will always be there to fulfil that physical and emotional need. I am certain that the physical closeness that nursing provides has helped her develop into the happy, smiling, laughing child that she is today.

Baby relaxes, mother relaxes. Breast-feeding has a tranquillizing effect on both mother and baby. After years of watching babies drift peacefully off to sleep at their mother's breast, we suspect that there is more at work here than the ambiance of baby's favourite "restaurant". Researchers have discovered a sleep-inducing protein in human milk, and we suspect that in years to come, many other baby-calming substances will be found in human milk. The needs of the frequent feeder force a mother to sit down and relax. In addition, hormones released during feedings have a soothing effect during a busy day. Breast-feeding has been known to put mothers, as well as babies, to sleep. Martha feels this is one physiologic source for getting the peace mothers need.

I tend to get overly committed and overly busy, and have always had a hard time budgeting my time and knowing my priorities. Breast-feeding our high-need child forced me to take time out, to relax, and put less important obligations on hold. Frequent breast-feeding gave me those extra five or ten times a day to just sit and caress, cuddle, and feed my baby, special times that passed all too soon. It's a tape I can't rewind and replay; I could enjoy it only for the moment. Breast-feeding made me realize other things can wait, as my baby has this special need only once in her life, and only once in my life do I have the privilege of meeting it.

problems mothers who breast-feed may encounter

While the hours you and your infant spend in touch with each other during feeding will be some of the most memorable moments of your life, there will be problems to solve along the way, especially with sensitive, high-need babies.

Nursing gymnastics. High-need babies are seldom still anywhere, even at the breast. Some squirm and arch their backs, and their tense little bodies may not mould into a comfortable feeding position, creating problems with latch-on and sucking. Improper latch-on is a common problem in the early weeks of breast-feeding, a problem that can be corrected early on (preferably in the first few days). You need to be shown how to take charge of your baby during feeding, bending her and moulding her to fit a correct feeding position. This encourages good latch-on and discourages her gymnastics. Feeding her in the baby sling can help keep her body curved and relaxed. One of the most frequent problems Martha has encountered in her lactation-counselling practice is the infant we dub "Little Tightmouth". Instead of latching on with a wide-open mouth, lips flanged open against the breast, some babies tend to purse and tighten their lips. They do not grasp enough of the breast to feed effectively, resulting in sore nipples and insufficient milk delivery. Work with your baby to get her to take the breast with a wide-open mouth. Once she has latched on, check the underside of the breast. If the lower lip is tucked in, a habit that causes a painful pinching sensation, correct it with what we call the "lower lip flip": With your index finger, depress baby's chin until the lower lip turns out underneath your breast. You may even need to do this (or have someone help) *while* baby is latching on to get the mouth open wider. (For more information about latch-on and sucking problems, contact NCT breast-feeding line 0870 444 8708 or Breast-feeding Network 0870 900 8787 or Association of breast-feeding mothers 0870 401 7711.)

Nursing distractions. "Little Miss Suck-a-Little, Look-a-Little" is now a few months old, so sensitive and distractible that she is on and off the breast many times during a feeding. Someone comes into the room, and she quickly turns her curious little head to see, taking your nipple right along with her. Try sheltered feeding with this baby. During the most distractible times of the day, feed your baby in a calm, quiet, darkened environment, such as your bedroom with curtains drawn. This change of environment minimizes distractions and acts as a cue to the baby, telling her that this is time to get down to the business of feeding and not playing.

Overenthusiastic feeding. High-need babies do everything more enthusiastically, even feed. Sometimes they will latch on ravenously and suck so fast that they swallow a lot of air, which can increase abdominal discomfort. Don't let baby get to the point of being ravenous; pay attention to the early, more subtle feeding cues so that he's more relaxed. If baby gets beside himself with impatience, his howling will cause him to swallow air even before the feeding starts (and it can cause you to tense up). All this air swallowing means less room in the stomach for milk, so you need to take time to burp this baby midway through each breast and when switching sides.

All-night nursing. Some mothers tell us that their high-need babies won't stay asleep unless they can stay attached to the breast the whole night. Why do some high-need babies do this? It could be because they are so needful of mother's presence that the only way they can "leave" her and go off to dreamland is if they can be certain she stays put. Or it could be that just as they do everything else intensely, they sleep intensely, too. As they suck off to sleep, the pressure generated in the mouth becomes part of their nighttime well-being. Anything that interrupts the pressure interrupts the sleep. High-need babies do not like to be rushed. If they are being hurried off the breast by a too-busy mum (or by a schedule that says only ten minutes per side), they react by hunkering down for the breast when they are less likely to be hurried. From the physical angle, night-long nursing can ease the internal irritation caused by food intolerance or the sensation of heartburn caused by gastroesophageal reflux (see pages 159–60). It's the one way baby knows to stay comfortable.

How to breast-feed lying down. If you expect to get any rest while baby is feeding all night, you need to master the side-lying position. It helps to have two pillows under your head (for having a better angle), a pillow behind your back, one under your top leg, and a fifth pillow to tuck behind baby. Five pillows may sound like a lot, but you need to be comfortable. Some babies like to rest their head on mum's arm, and some babies like to lie on the mattress next to mum. Some mothers find that once baby is older and heavier, their arms go to sleep from the pressure on them, so you'll have to experiment with what works best for you. You'll also have to find the right angle to line baby's mouth up with your nipple. Once the two of you find your favourite side-lying position, sleep will be a lot easier. Martha found that keeping a night-light on helped the night-feeding process by providing just enough light to see what she was doing without waking the baby up. (The night-light also helped her change nappies in the dark.)

After a few weeks of using the Moses basket at night, I decided it was time to learn the side-lying approach to breast-feeding because I was getting exhausted. It took us at least a week or two before we were able to do this at all. We had many challenges. Philip often couldn't latch on because he couldn't find my nipple in the dark. He would latch on for a minute and then come off, and we had to relatch all over again. This situation was waking my husband and even my visiting mother in the other room for many nights. Philip and I persisted, and after a few weeks it became less difficult. The side-lying position was important for me, because it allowed me to rest while Philip nursed several times at night.

Tips on solving the all-night feeding problem.
One way to change this behaviour is to get baby to go to sleep without sucking. Breast-feed long enough to give baby a good feed, and then stop the feeding and rock, walk, or dance him off to sleep. To transition baby down to where he sleeps will require some creativity, especially if he sleeps in a cot. If he sleeps in your bed, you can just lie with him in your arms (but not attached!) until you can sneak away or fall asleep yourself. This whole process may take longer to get him down, but at least you'll be free until he wakes the first time.

However, high-need babies seem to wake sooner if no one is next to them, and sleep-association theory (that is, the person or prop that baby associates with falling asleep) says that babies who go to sleep at the breast will need the breast to get back to sleep. This may be truer of older babies who have had time to develop a system for themselves. Very young babies will usually need to feed when they wake up, regardless of how they were put down. So the next time baby wakes, be willing to spend the time walking, rocking, or dancing again, proceeded by a breast-feed if he's slept long enough to be hungry. And who's to say how long that is? This is a lot of physical and mental gymnastics to be doing in the middle of the night, with or without some verbal accompaniment from baby. Who can blame mothers for taking the easy way out and just pulling baby over and giving him the breast when he wakes? So now you're back to square one: baby is (back to) sleeping, but won't let go of your breast.

Here's how Martha solved this problem after she found out the hard way that Hayden would startle awake as soon as Martha slipped her nipple out of Hayden's mouth.

Being high-need myself (really needing to get her off my breast so I could get some time to myself or get to sleep), I kept experimenting until I came up with what worked. I discovered that if I got my nipple free while still maintaining the feeling of pressure in her mouth, Hayden would stay asleep. To do this, take hold of your breast in a C-hold thumb on top of breast and fingers under. Carefully ease your nipple away after breaking suction. (Experiment with doing this very quickly or very gradually.)

Immediately put pressure under baby's chin or lower lip with your index finger, pressing upward and inward as soon as your nipple clears the jaws. Hold the pressure steady until baby settles back to deep sleep. If baby rouses completely and grasps for the "lost" nipple, let her have it, and try again after she's sucked back to a deep sleep. You may have to do this several times before baby stays asleep, but it often works on the first try if baby is deep enough in sleep and you have been patient enough not to rush it.

Constant feeding. Remember the trademark of high-need babies: more. They want to feed *more*. They feed longer, stronger, and more often. "My baby wants to feed all day and night" is a complaint of tired mothers. While all babies occasionally "marathon feed" during growth spurts, this seems to be the predominant pattern for high-need babies. Most babies change their feeding pattern between three and six months of age, and begin to feed more frequently during the day and less frequently at night. High-need babies often feed as frequently during the night as they do during the day. As they get older, they become so busy with other activities during the day that they forget to feed, and, of course, they need to make up for these missed feeds during the night. If your baby is going through one of these marathon feeding stages (and most do), try these tips:

Create a feeding station. Set up a calm, quiet, attractive area, complete with a supportive place to sit (perhaps a rocking chair or a couch corner), where you can stuff pillows and place snacks and beverages on an adjacent table; a footstool; pleasant music (preferably with a remote control), a phone nearby (or off the hook); and your favourite novel, joke books, or whatever can help keep you amused. Arrange this "nest" to meet your needs during these frequent feeding times so that you can meet the needs of your baby.

Tank up baby during the day. For the baby who feeds frequently during the night but less often during the day, step in and take charge of her feeding pattern. Feed her frequently during the day, at least every two or three hours. A newborn will often sleep most of the day if you let her, only to be awake much of the night. For the older baby, try sheltered feeding, as mentioned above, by finding a place in your home that is conducive to baby settling down to feed while you relax. The earlier baby gets the message that nighttime is for sleeping and daytime is for feeding and playing, the more all of you will sleep. Some babies do not seem to get this message on their own; they have to be taught. Some mothers who share sleep with their baby can feed a lot at night and still get sufficient rest; they enjoy these special private night feeds. Other mothers wake up feeling exhausted after feeding every one to two hours; this makes it difficult to be an effective parent during the day. In our experience, "Don't worry, he'll grow out of it" is not helpful advice for exhausted mothers of frequent night-feeders. True, babies do grow out of it, but it may take years. In feeding, as in all aspects of infant behaviour, parents have to participate in shaping their infant's habits. You can't change your baby's temperament or her need level, but you can gently teach her better ways to behave. Of course, during stressful times (e.g., illness, teething, or a change in family routine), babies' nighttime needs intensify, and they need to be met. (Also see Chapter 10, "Hidden Causes of Fussiness in Infants".)

Indefinite feeding. High-need babies not only feed more frequently and more intensely, they breast-feed for a longer time. While our culture usually measures breast-feeding duration in months, high-need babies usually log a few years at the breast. These smart babies realize they have a good thing going, and they're not about to give it up. Early weaning is not recommended for any babies, and especially not for high-need ones. Many people in our misguided culture are shocked by the sight of a breast-feeding toddler. Yet, in many other cultures, breast-feeding for several years is the norm, and recent evidence suggests that it is a healthy norm.

Extended breast-feeding is not only the preference of the high-need toddler, it's a lifesaver for the mother. Breast-feeding is one of the most useful comforting tools available to a mother during transition stages when high-need children intensify their behaviour to show their higher needs. Mothers use nursing to avoid tantrums, to soothe ouchies, to settle the resistant napper, to resettle the frequent waker, and to quiet a disturbing toddler.

Criticisms. At some time during your breast-feeding experience, expect a poorly informed adviser to exclaim "What? You're still feeding?" and to offer one or more of the following criticisms:

- "You're making her so dependent." Non-sense. You are nurturing your child in a way that helps her learn to trust herself and others; this will help her achieve healthy independence. In our experience of following hundreds of extended nursers, these babies become independent and well-adjusted children. Our highest-need, and now quite independent child, Hayden, weaned at four years. Our other self-weaners did so between three and three and a half years.
- "You're doing it for yourself." While many mothers enjoy feeding their toddler, the child's needs take preference. A toddler who is ready to wean or cut back on feedings will do so, and while mothers may feel a certain sadness at weaning, most also find joy in the way the child easily moves on to the next stage.
- "He's manipulating you." A nursing toddler is communicating a need and you are responding to that need. This is not manipulation; it's communication, and it's healthy. The trust and comfort toddlers find in breast-feeding helps them as they struggle to learn what they may and may not do. Parents of extended feeders often find the "terrible twos" to be a myth. Remember, though, that you're in charge of the feeding. You can choose whether or not to feed, and it's okay to say "not now" or "later" if the situation warrants it. A toddler will not be devastated emotionally by being frustrated the way an infant would be.

When is it time to wean? There is no simple answer to this question. Weaning is an interactive process; it involves both members of the breast-feeding pair. The child's stage of development, the mother's willingness to feed, and what's happening in the family all influence weaning. Mother might choose to help the process along a little by avoiding a favourite nursing chair, and the fun of playing outside in the summer or going to a playgroup will make a child less interested in breast-feeding. A mother who feels she needs to wean her toddler should think carefully about her situation. Feeling that you need to wean is often symptomatic of some other need, perhaps some time for yourself or a desire for a better body image. Weaning may not meet the real need. But if your need to wean is overwhelming (see "Time to Move On", page 253), be confident that you can continue your attachment in other ways as your toddler grows toward individuation.

"Weaning" is not a negative term. It is not the loss of a relationship, but rather a passage from one stage to another. Weaning means that a child is *filled*, filled with one relationship, and because of that fulfilment, ready to take on other relationships. In ancient Hebrew writings the word for weaning also meant "to ripen", the same word used when a fruit was ripe and ready to be picked from the vine. When the child was ready to wean, the community got together and celebrated, not because the mother was finally free of the clingy child, but because the child was now ripe and ready to take on new relationships. Weaning was a festive occasion. There is a calmness and fulfilment associated with the concept of weaning, the image of a weaned child in a state of peace and tranquillity as so beautifully written by the Psalmist:

I have stilled and quieted my soul, like a weaned child with its mother, like a weaned child is my soul within me.

high-need stage

The age of fourteen to eighteen months is a very demanding one, with a lot of energy required from mum. If a child's needs continue to be met during this time, then the weanings that come along after eighteen months will be emotionally easier for the parent and the child. Attachment during this high-need stage fills a deep need for staying calm. It provides a spiritual nourishment vital to his well-being, much as breast-feeding and being carried a lot nurtured him physically during the first year. Get through this high-need stage by recognizing and responding to the intensity of it, then look forward to the weanings ahead without anxiety.

formula-feeding fussy babies

Allergy to formula ranks high on the list of medical causes of infant colic. Even though I am not aware of any studies on the incidence of allergies among high-need babies, it's my general impression that these infants are more prone to food- and formula-sensitivities. Perhaps the overall super-sensitivity that affects their behaviour also influences their food tolerances. So, if you are unable to breast-feed or choose not to, choosing the right formula for your baby may take some extra care. Here are some time-tested ways of formula-feeding high-need babies.

Start early. If you or your partner has a family history of milk- or formula-sensitivity, or if your other children were allergic to milk or certain formulas, alert your baby's doctor or health visitor to these facts. Your doctor may advise you to start your baby on a hypoallergenic formula right after birth, before waiting for colicky symptoms to appear.

Choose the right formula. Based upon your wishes and your baby's medical needs, your health visitor and GP will help you choose the right formula to begin feeding your baby. There are three basic types of formula from which to choose for feeding your infant during the first year:

1. milk-based formulas, those with cow's milk as the protein base
2. soy formulas, using soybean as the protein source. These do not contain the milk sugar lactose
3. hypoallergenic formulas, those in which the protein has been made less allergenic

Unless there is a medical reason to the contrary, most paediatricians prefer milk-based formulas. These have a longer track record, and there are more studies on their safety. Soy itself is a common allergen, and approximately 35 per cent of infants who are allergic to cow's milk are also allergic to soy. I am concerned about the absence of lactose in soy formulas and most hypoallergenic formulas. Many nutritionists suspect that lactose is a necessary nutrient for the infant's rapidly developing brain. Also, the corn syrup that substitutes for lactose is in itself a potential allergen. Another consideration is the taste and cost of special formulas. As the allergenicity of the formulas goes down, the price goes up, and the taste gets worse. The most hypoallergenic formulas are quite expensive (although being available on prescription there may be a subsidy) and somewhat unpalatable, causing some taste-sensitive infants to refuse them.

Watch for signs of formula allergies. Babies who are allergic to formula have one or more of the following symptoms:

- bursts of crying, abdominal pain, and vomiting right after feeding
- explosive, mucusy diarrhoea
- a painful, tense, bloated abdomen
- a generally irritable baby
- frequent night waking
- frequent colds and/or ear infections
- a red, raised, sandpaper-like rash on the cheeks and/or around the anus

In my experience, if babies are truly allergic to or intolerant of any milk or food, they have more than just behavioural symptoms; expect to see a rash on the face, runny nose, colicky behaviour, abdominal pain, or diarrhoea.

Minimize air swallowing. A key to feeding enthusiastic high-need babies is to get the most formula in with the least amount of air. Check the baby's position on the teat to make sure the baby is making a good seal all the way around. Experiment with various types of holding, burping, teats, and bottles until you and your baby have worked out the most comfortable feeding. These preferences may change as your baby grows.

Offer small, frequent feedings. Before you begin the whole formula-switching circus, try offering your baby smaller feedings more frequently, perhaps half as much twice as often. Some infants, especially those who suffer bloating from lactose overload, can digest smaller volumes without intestinal discomfort.

Make feeding time nurturing time. Remember, infant feeding, whether by breast or by bottle, is a time for social interaction, in addition to providing nutrition. Hold your baby lovingly during feeding; caress and interact with your baby. Some babies feed better when you're quiet, but they still need your loving presence. Don't prop the bottle and walk away. When babies begin to walk resist the temptation to let them walk away with the bottle – it will make for a calmer toddler and easier bottle-weaning later. Remember, there should always be a person at both ends of the bottle.

high needs – high nutrition

While many food scientists doubt the relationship between what children eat and how they behave, mothers of high-need children swear a food-mood connection exists. Sensitivity to certain foods seems to be part of a high-need child's overall hypersensitivity to everything.

Encourage nutrient-dense foods. These are foods that are packed with a lot of nutrition in a small volume of food. Nutrient-dense foods are particularly important for the picky eater who doesn't eat a great deal. You want to make every calorie count. Nutrient-dense foods include avocado, brown rice, cheese, egg, fish, kidney beans, whole-grain pasta, tofu, and turkey. You can make these foods more appealing by giving your child a favourite sauce in which to dip them. Stephen's favourite is creamy Italian salad dressing.

Eliminate bad-behaviour foods. These are foods that either excite an already excitable child, such as some food colourings and caffeine, or produce a roller-coaster effect on the child's blood-sugar level and corresponding mood swings, such as sugars that enter the bloodstream fast and are used up quickly. Some children go "hyper" on corn syrup, the main ingredient in sweets and soft drinks; other foods to avoid include table sugar, glucose, sucrose, dextrose, and brown sugar; these are found in large amounts in sweets, icing, soft drinks, and many cereals. Since sugars normally provide at least half of a healthy child's energy needs, it's important to concentrate on sugars that do not cause such blood-sugar swings because they take longer to digest. These include the fructose in fruit and the lactose in dairy products. Best of all for behaviour and good health are complex carbohydrates, or what granny called starches. These are like time-release sugars that enter and leave the bloodstream more slowly. They include whole-grain breads and crackers, pasta, unsweetened cereals, rice, and other grains. These are especially valuable for children who burn calories as fast as they eat them. Whether sugar affects your child's behaviour can be determined only by trial and error.

Food sensitivities can affect a child's behaviour at any age. Even though living with our daughter Hayden got easier as she got older, we had to be constantly aware of things that might affect her behaviour. For example, when Hayden was eight years old, she would sometimes burst into fits of rage at the slightest provocation, wearing down the nerves of everyone around her. By doing some detective work we found her fits stopped when we eliminated corn and corn syrup from her diet. (For more information see "Food Sensitivities", page 155.)

grazing

High-energy children burn a lot of calories. This explains why their behaviour often deteriorates just before lunch and dinner. One of the ways to mellow the moods of high-need children is to encourage them to feed frequently. Grazing stabilizes blood-sugar levels, preventing the mood swings that occur when children go more than a few hours without food.

Actually, all young children do better grazing all day than being asked to sit down and eat "three squares" and being urged to eat more than they want of food their body doesn't need. Research on toddlers showed that over a period of thirty days, they chose a balanced diet, though some days it was just raisins and bread, other days vegetables and rice, and others just fruit. Pushing food only creates eating disorders later.

One of the ways we smooth the roller-coaster behaviour of our children is to make it easy for them to graze frequently on nutritious snacks. For the toddler, we prepare a nibble tray: an ice cube tray filled with nutritious, bite-size, nutrient-dense foods, such as pieces of cheese, hard-boiled egg wedges, bread strips, pasta pieces, and bite-size fruits and vegetables. We fill one or two compartments with a nutritious dip, such as guacamole or yoghurt sweetened with fruit only. We place the nibble tray on the toddler's own table, where he can sit and graze as needed. For the older child, we make snacks easily available in the pantry or refrigerator. To get more mileage out of your nibble trays and snacks, let your child select nutritious snacks at the supermarket and help you prepare the trays.

chapter 10

hidden causes of
fussiness in infants

Even the most experienced parents and astute doctors can be fooled by the healthy appearance of a high-need baby and miss an underlying medical cause for baby's extreme behaviour.

- Baby has periodic sudden outbursts of inconsolable crying, as if in pain.
- Baby awakens shrieking as if in pain and is difficult to resettle without feeding.
- Older baby is unable to sleep at least one three-hour stretch at night.
- Nothing works; baby is not getting better.
- Your intuition tells you your baby hurts somewhere.

A pain in the gut can be as simple to relieve as changing the way you close baby's nappy. Some sensitive little midsections cannot stomach (pun intended) constriction. A mother discovered this when she got severe abdominal cramping from a tight waistband. The following are the most common medical causes of colicky crying in young babies (less than six months old) and night waking in older babies (more than six months).

While baby's reaction to emotional pain can mimic physical discomfort, here are some general guidelines for when to suspect a physical cause for baby's fussiness:

food sensitivities

New research is confirming what old wives have long suspected: food- and formula-sensitivities can cause colicky behaviour in babies. Suspect a sensitivity to formula or to something in your breast milk if any of the following are true:

- Baby's fussiness escalates or colicky pain occurs within minutes to an hour after feeding.
- Baby seems gassy or bloated after feeding.
- Baby possets frequently soon after feeding.
- Baby begins to breast-feed but keeps pulling off, crying as if in pain. (The irritated gut starts churning during a feeding, which can make every feeding time quite unpleasurable for the sensitive/allergic baby and quite frustrating for mothers.)

is it colic?

Most high-need babies were sometime in their early lives labelled "colicky". The point at which a "fussy baby" or "high need baby" becomes a "colicky baby" is often a matter of interpretation, and what you call the baby's situation is nowhere near as meaningful as what you do about it. In paediatric practice I have found it helpful to use the term "high need baby" when I suspect that it is the baby's temperament causing the behaviour and "colic" when suspecting a medical reason. Colicky babies hurt. They don't merely fuss; they shriek in agonizing discomfort. "Colicky" calls for a different approach than "high-need".

Our daughter, now thirteen months, was the queen of colic. She'd start at three o'clock and cry non-stop till about midnight. When she wasn't being colicky, she was just plain high-need. There IS a difference! "High-need" responds to attachment parenting; almost nothing works for colic!

If you suspect colic, in partnership with your doctor or health visitor, keep searching for a medical or physical reason for why your baby hurts. I advise parents to use the term "hurting baby" instead of "colicky baby", as this label will better motivate everyone to uncover the cause. For a thorough step-by-step method of diagnosing and comforting colic consult *The Baby Book* (Thorsons, 2005).

- Baby shows a change in bowel habits (either infrequent stools or diarrhoea).
- Baby's bowel movements are extremely watery, mucusy, or explosive.
- Baby shows what we call the "target sign": a red, circular rash around the anus caused by the skin reacting to irritating bowel movements.
- Baby has frequent ear infections.
- Baby's sleep is restless and fitful, waking every ninety minutes (or less!), or baby can stay asleep only with mum's nipple in her mouth.
- Baby cries with night waking and cannot be easily parented back to sleep.
- Baby shows an obvious change in behaviour following a change in mother's diet.
- Baby may not be thriving. Most infants with an underlying medical condition serious enough to cause severe pain usually do not gain weight normally or have that well-baby appearance. (This is only a general correlation and is not always true. Some infants with hidden medical causes of colic can be the picture of perfect health.)

Problems may also start at the time solid food is introduced. Babies with food intolerance typically are late to eat solids.

If you are breast-feeding, here's how to uncover hidden food sensitivities:

Make a diary of possible fuss foods. List the foods you have eaten most frequently in the past week, especially those you particularly enjoy or tend to "overdose" on. Also list any unusual foods you have eaten in the past few days, foods you would not ordinarily eat.

List baby's most bothersome behaviours.

Try an elimination diet. In addition to those suspect foods in your diary, eliminate the following most common "fuss foods" from your diet for at least two weeks, either one each week until they are all eliminated or all at once:

- dairy products (remember to take a calcium supplement). Besides milk this includes: yoghurt, ice cream, cheese, butter, and products with the words whey, casein, and sodium caseinate on their labels. It is important to read ingredient labels because milk or its protein derivatives, whey and casein, are added to many foods, such as bread, sausages, salad dressings, margarine, soups, chocolate, and so on.
- nuts and peanut butter
- corn
- caffeine (cola, coffee, tea – one serving a day)

Less common fuss foods in a breast-feeding mother's diet are wheat, egg white, shellfish, citrus, tomato, apple juice, soy, and gassy vegetables (raw cabbage, broccoli, cauliflower, peppers, onions, beans), and many spices.

Is there a correlation? Do you see an obvious change in your baby's behaviour following elimination of certain foods? Words of caution:

Be objective. In your desperation to comfort your baby, it's easy to pin the blame on food sensitivity. You are willing to try anything, and your desire for a solution can cloud your objectivity. It may take several weeks to identify an offending food, and by that time simple maturity could improve your baby's behaviour. Most mothers are so delighted when their baby feels better that they are not very exacting about proving the cause-and-effect relationship. If you want to be more objective and scientific about your elimination diet (and avoid depriving yourself unnecessarily of needed or wanted foods), retry the suspected offending food once or twice and see if the behaviour recurs.

Be nutritionally wise. A nutrient-deprived mother and a high-need baby make an exhausting match. While it's not difficult to eliminate a short list of foods without depriving yourself of needed nutrients, a multi-food elimination diet for more than two weeks would be unwise without nutritional counselling. You must continue to feed yourself right in order to care for your baby and yourself. (See "An Elimination Diet", page 158.)

Consider the threshold effect. A small amount of some foods may not bother baby in the way large quantities do. This is especially true of dairy products. For example, some babies get colicky if the mother "overdoses" on a pint of milk a day but are not bothered if mother enjoys an occasional yoghurt shake.

I drank apricot juice almost daily during my pregnancy, and my daughter Beth (now eight years old) is still allergic to it. My friend Susan was given a case of popcorn and she snacked on it several times a day until it ran out at about three weeks postpartum. After this, she had to cut way back on all corn products for about nine months, and then began to very slowly introduce them into her diet again.

• • •

an elimination diet

This is a diet that Martha recommends whenever she suspects a baby's colic or frequent night waking could be caused by sensitivities to food in a breast-feeding mother's diet. This type of diet has several variations, depending on how severe the symptoms are. The elimination diet we use is based on eating the least troublesome food in each of the food groups. You may need to do this for two weeks, since it can take this long for the offending foods to get out of your system and baby's system. Here is the variation we find helps mothers get the quickest, surest relief for their hurting babies:

- Eat only turkey and lamb, baked or boiled potatoes and sweet potatoes (with salt and pepper only), rice and millet as your only grain, cooked courgette, marrow or pumpkin for your vegetable, and for fruit, pears and diluted pear juice. (If you are desperate for variety, try poi, probably the least allergenic food there is.) Use a rice-based beverage to drink and in place of milk on cereal or in cooking. Do not use soy beverages. Take a calcium supplement. (Rice products, such as rice beverages, rice-based frozen desserts, rice pasta, rice flour, and millet, are available in health food stores.) Free range turkey and lamb are best. Read labels, as suggested on page 157.

- At the end of two weeks, or sooner if the colic subsides, gradually add other foods to your diet, one every four days, starting with those less commonly offending (such as sunflower seeds, carrots, lettuce, salmon, barley, grapes, avocado, and peaches), and watch for the effects on your baby. Wait for a while before you add wheat, chicken, beef, eggs, nuts, and corn. Avoid for the longest time dairy products, soy products, peanuts, shellfish, coffee, tea, colas and other beverages containing caffeine, chocolate, gas-producing vegetables (broccoli, cauliflower, cabbage, onions, and green peppers), tomatoes, and citrus fruits. Vegetables and fruits are often tolerated in cooked form sooner than in raw form.
- Keep a record of the foods you eat and the problem behaviours; try to correlate baby's fussy spells with what you've eaten in the past day or so. This gives you a clearer perspective and helps you stay objective, which is hard to do when you are sleep-deprived. This is especially important when baby has stayed fussy past four months of age.

Do not starve yourself. It may feel, the first day or two, as though there is not enough for you to eat; but you can still eat a nutritious diet. You just have to eat more of the "safe" types of food until you determine what your baby can tolerate.

Colicky babies usually respond to mother's diet changes dramatically and quickly, often within one or two days. With the older baby for whom the main symptom of food sensitivities is night waking, you may have to wait longer to see results. Typically, mothers will find that when they change their diet, baby may sleep better for a few nights only to start waking frequently again for a few days or a week, at which time the sleep again improves. It's important to know this so that you will not be tempted to give up when you think it's not working.

Older babies are often less sensitive to fruits and vegetables in mum's diet (and their own), so at this stage we recommend mainly protein elimination, namely dairy, beef, eggs, chicken, shellfish, soy, corn, wheat, and peanuts (plus any other foods you have learned bother baby). Research has shown that some foreign proteins get into some mothers' milk more than others, and of course some babies are more sensitive to these proteins than other babies.

For additional information on food sensitivities, see the mothers' stories on pages 233 and 238–9.

I began a food diary. I was not willing to allow my baby to suffer. I watched for skin changes, particularly the "allergic ring" around her anus. This was very helpful. My baby would get an oval redness around her anus when I ate something that would bother her and make her cry. A baby's bowel movement should not burn her skin. (I change her nappy very frequently, so I knew that the redness was not nappy rash!) Her bottom would get very red within hours of the offending food. I worked out that dairy, oats, and corn can affect my baby immensely. Since I've eliminated these foods, the crying has stopped and she is a different baby.

Most infants outgrow their food sensitivities within the first year or two, and their breast-feeding mothers can eventually enjoy a bountiful diet without causing fussiness in their babies. However, I have discovered there are many older high-need children whose behaviour is still affected by food sensitivities. In fact, food sensitivities can affect a child's behaviour at any age.

Some mothers have found that by simply removing themselves from stressful situations or by avoiding adrenaline-producing situations, their babies' digestive tracts and nervous systems settle down. It's worth considering slowing down and backing off from the rat race before devoting yourself to a restrictive diet.

gastroesophageal reflux

Gastroesophageal reflux (GER) is a recently identified medical problem that masquerades as colic. In this condition the stomach contracts and regurgitates irritating acids into the

looks are deceiving

Extreme mood swings in high-need babies can mimic colicky behaviour. Both colicky and high-need babies behave at times like Dr Jekyll and Mr Hyde. One minute baby is the picture of contentment; the next minute she's an emotional wreck. Most colicky babies, especially those for whom there appears to be no underlying medical cause, appear to be the picture of good health. Onlookers remark, "My, what a healthy-looking baby. You're so lucky." The drained mother responds, "You should have seen us an hour ago."

oesophagus, resulting in the kind of pain adults call heartburn. Clues that your baby may suffer from reflux are:

- colicky abdominal signs after eating: baby draws up knees to abdomen, writhes or grimaces as if in pain
- painful bursts of night waking, quickly soothed by feeding
- posseting during or shortly after feeding (In some babies, the acidic spit-up comes only partway up the oesophagus, far enough to cause pain but not far enough to see.)
- frequent, unexplained stop-breathing episodes, wheezing, or lung infections

Babies with GER show less colicky behaviour when carried upright, allowing gravity to hold the stomach contents down. However, babies generally settle when carried, regardless of the cause of the colic, so don't interpret this behaviour

as diagnostic of GER. If your parent's intuition suggests that your baby is truly hurting, ask your doctor to investigate for GER. Babies with GER are soothed remarkably well by medications that neutralize the stomach acids and empty the stomach more quickly. You can also elevate the head of baby's cot mattress at a 30 degree angle to keep baby upright as much as possible when sleeping. Breast-feed as often and as long as possible. GER occurs less frequently and less severely in breast-feeding infants. Consult a paediatric gastro-enterologist who is especially knowledgeable about the diagnosis and treatment of GER. In my paediatric experience, I have found that GER is a common hidden cause of so-called colic and painful night waking. (See a mother's story about her baby with GER, pages 229–33.)

a pain in the gut

As you keep searching for physical causes of your baby's fussiness, consider the intestinal tract as the most likely site. From the top to the bottom of the intestines, the possible causes of colic are gastro-oesophageal reflux, food sensitivities, constipation, and a cause that receives little attention – a tight rectal opening, which prevents easy passage of bowel movements. (Dr David Sharp of the Sharp Colic Clinic in Grand Rapids, Michigan, has reported relieving many babies of colic after he performs a finger dilation of the procedure enabling easier passage of stools.) If your baby is not just fussy but is really hurting, keep searching – ask your doctor about these possible intestinal causes of your baby's pain.

ear infections

Children who don't feel well don't act well. This is true at all ages. The pressure of infected fluid on an inflamed eardrum can cause an infant or child to become irritable, especially when he is lying down. Sinus infections often accompany ear infections, further aggravating the child's discomfort and behaviour. Some children don't act sick with ear and sinus infections, they just get irritable and cranky. Here are the clues that an underlying ear infection may be affecting your child's behaviour:

- frequent colds that progress to a yellow-green discharge from the nose
- yellow drainage from the corners of the eyes near the nose
- peaked facial appearance (pale face, puffy eyelids, dark circles under eyes)
- frequent night waking from pain
- tiredness

Have your doctor check the ears and sinuses of your older child too if they exhibit these symptoms.

anaemia

Anaemia, or a low red blood-cell count, can cause irritable behaviour in babies older than nine months. The most common cause of anaemia in infants and children is iron deficiency. Iron is needed to make red blood cells. Clues that your child may be iron deficient include the following:

a sample "fuss food" detection exercise

Possible Fuss Foods	Fussy Behaviours
dairy products, nuts, corn	frequent, painful night wakings, frequent outbursts of abdominal pain – especially after feeding

Foods Eliminated	Behaviour Changes
nuts	no difference detected
dairy products	slept better, seemed less colicky

never stop looking for answers

Features	High-Need Baby (fussy baby)	Colicky Baby (hurting baby)
Intense crying	settles when held, consolable	shrieks inconsolably
Behaviour pattern	no consistent pattern	painful outbursts interspersed with periods of calmness; usually occurs in late afternoon and evening; alternating periods of contentment and violent outbursts: "He seemed perfectly happy and content just a minute ago. Now he's a wreck, and so are we."
Body language and facial features	upset, a fretful look, tense muscles, often relaxes when held	"ouch" signs: facial grimaces, furrowed forehead, crying with wide-open mouth, clenched fists, hard tummy, flailing arms and legs, arms clenched tightly to chest and knees drawn up against a bloated abdomen, back arching, brief post-colicky snooze as if "spent"
Parents' intuition	"It's her temperament."	"I know he hurts somewhere."

At three weeks of age Lea became very fussy and cried all day long. She would awaken in the morning fussing, and by late afternoon it would turn into an unreachable screaming and crying fit – unreachable because there was no way to calm her down and she seemed totally unaware of her surroundings. Her eyes were open but she did not see. Her crying was very loud and her whole face would turn red, and I often thought she was going to stop breathing. During the day, she fed very infrequently and only for a few minutes if she did at all. She would latch onto the breast and after a few sucks throw her head back, arch her back, and start screaming. It was nearly impossible to get her to sleep during the day, and transitioning from wakefulness to sleep was very difficult for her.

My mother-in-law, who had the same problem with one of her babies (in fact, it was Matthew – Bill and Martha Sears's sixth baby), told me to do what she did: "Go on an elimination diet for two to three weeks (see page 158)." Lea's colic improved greatly within two days.

I do believe that in some way all of this has made me more "attached" to my daughter, and I think I will be a more sensitive and responsive parent because of it. I never let her cry it out and I never stopped looking for answers, and I probably never will.

- pale skin, most noticeable in the earlobes
- suspected deficiency of iron in child's diet (drinks a lot of milk or low-iron formula, but eats few iron-fortified foods)
- history of milk- or formula-allergy (this increases loss of blood and iron from irritated intestinal lining)

As part of routine well-baby care, your doctor will measure your baby's haemoglobin between nine and twelve months.

urinary tract infections

A urinary tract infection (UTI) is a rare but potentially serious cause of colic if left untreated.

Infants with urinary tract infections serious enough to cause colicky behaviour usually (but not always) show other symptoms, such as

- unexplained fevers
- poor growth
- unexplained vomiting
- abdominal pain

"Colic" that doesn't go away and is otherwise unexplained should raise the suspicion of a possible underlying urinary tract infection. A doctor should investigate.

The cause of baby's crying and/or night waking can be as simple and obvious as teething, as strange as pinworms, as puzzling as food or environmental sensitivities, or as elusive as problems in basic body chemistry, which,

thank you for not smoking

Babies whose parents or caregivers smoke are more likely to be colicky for a variety of reasons. Nicotine and other chemicals in cigarette smoke pass into baby's bloodstream (either through breast milk or by second-hand smoke) and may act as behavioural irritants. Smoke irritates a baby's sensitive breathing passages, clogging them with mucus and predisposing the child to ear and sinus infections and the miserable behaviour that accompanies them.

Not only do babies of smoking parents fuss more but smoking mothers may be less able to cope with a fussy baby. Research shows that mothers who smoke have lower levels of prolactin, the mothering hormone that helps a mother feel relaxed and more sensitive to her baby. Smoking and childcare don't mix, especially for high-need children.

If it is unrealistic for a mother to quit smoking, she can find strategies that help her cut way down on the number of cigarettes she smokes and never smoke in her baby's presence. Best is to smoke outdoors, so the fumes and chemicals don't accumulate in the household furnishings.

while rare, do happen. Here are two mothers' stories:

It turned out my baby had a urinary tract infection last week. To calm her crying I was up feeding her for several nights. I knew something was wrong with her and I finally took her to the doctor. If I had taken other people's advice – that she was manipulating me and I should let her cry it out – I would not have been in tune with her and would have delayed having her checked. This experience was a real validation of attachment parenting.

• • •

We were desperate about our baby, Anna. I wasn't willing to accept the doctor's diagnosis that, as a two-year-old, she was "neurologically impaired" and "emotionally disturbed" just because she cried all the time. I knew she was in constant pain, but no doctor could help her. Somehow we found the strength to keep searching. We were convinced there was help out there. We went from specialist to specialist: a neurologist, a paediatrician-nutritionist, a paediatric gastro-enterologist, and we even took her to one of the best children's hospitals in the country, where she had her own team of specialists. All of these doctors gave us different pieces of the puzzle, finally putting it together as a problem in her blood chemistry, which she had been born with: extremely high calcium, low iron and other mineral deficiencies, and an extreme intolerance to sorbitol (a natural sugar found in apples, grapes, cherries, and pears), all of which interfered with her sleep and caused distorted muscle function of her gastrointestinal tract. After dietary treatment, she became a happy, healthy little girl. I'm glad we didn't just accept that she was "colicky" and that "some babies just cry all the time" and that we didn't stop searching for answers.

II

the high-need child grows up

High-need babies grow up to be high-need children, and how you parent your infant will set the stage for how you parent your growing child. In Part 1, we presented the concept of high-need infants and ways to respond sensitively to their needs. While the high-maintenance and physically draining stage of parenting is behind you, the emotionally draining yet exciting stage lies ahead. Needs don't get less as children get older, they simply change. In this part of the book we will talk about learning to live with high-need children, how to take charge of them before they take charge of you, and how to discipline and relate to challenging children who will bring out your best communication skills.

chapter 11

the high-need thrill ride

In counselling parents with high-need children and in preparation for writing this book, we asked many parents to write us their stories. The quotes from these letters have been used throughout this book to add insight into and examples of what we have described. Reading these letters has been helpful to us, and writing them has been therapeutic for the parents.

This exercise helped them make sense of where they've been and where they're headed. This entire chapter is an account of one mother's experiences with her high-need children.

the ride begins

You fasten the strap across your lap, making certain it's tight enough, and your heart starts beating faster in anticipation. The operator walks by to check that the belt is secure and then returns to the control booth. Your heart beats even faster as he throws the switch, and your car lurches into a slow movement. Up, up a hill, slowly, *slooooowly* – suddenly you're at the top, and you go plunging down and around in a wild, spinning swoop that makes your stomach drop,

and you're not sure the track will ever level out. But it does, and you no sooner catch your breath than you're off on another plunge. Maybe you scream, or shout, but you find it difficult as the wind rushing past blows your hair back and stifles the noise before it leaves your mouth.

It sounds like torture, but most of us love a roller coaster! Soon the ride ends, and you may even say, "Let's go again!" Still, a few times are enough, and it's time to return to level ground. I like a good, scary roller-coaster ride as much as the next person, but I wouldn't choose to ride one *all* the time. Would you?

Children are a bit like roller coasters. They enter our lives, and we know the track won't be entirely smooth. It will have its ups and downs, and at times our stomachs will drop. Having a high-need child, however, is more like being strapped into the roller coaster all the time. Just when you think the ride is over, or at least that the track has levelled off, your child finds a way to take you on another stomach-churning twist. It's hard to get your equilibrium. You just want *off* for a while!

But if you as a parent can learn to strap yourself in tight for the bumpy times, the ride can be thrilling … and very rewarding. And eventually it does end. It just won't end on your schedule. Count on it.

"Don't I have any control?" you may wonder. Well, yes. The roller coaster analogy only goes so far. The high-need child needs all the things other children need; she just needs them in higher doses. She is determined to find ways to get what she needs, where other children might simply do without and perhaps suffer for it. If she can't get those needs met, she'll suffer too, but she'll do it in spectacular ways that will make others suffer right along with her. Your best option for control is to find ways to fulfil those needs and make life easier for everyone.

Are you surrendering your rightful parental authority to a problem child? Some people think so, and I would have too – before I had a high-need child. But I've come to realize that meeting a genuine need is not surrendering: it's responsible parenting, in recognition of the uniqueness of each child. It's very different from granting a child's every want, and it must be coupled with responsible discipline.

It's also very important to realize that having a high-need child is not a negative thing! Challenges in our lives (and a high-need child is definitely a challenge!) make us strong. They force us to evaluate, sort out, refocus, and dedicate ourselves to what really counts, to eliminate what's unimportant and concentrate on what's important. The high-need child will help you mature right along with him. Believe me!

The parenting ride is different with every child, and high-need children are no exception. Every child is unique, and no one high-need child has all the so-called high-need traits. We have three sons; Harry and Tom, now almost grown, and Charlie, now well into school. We were blessed with two high-need children among the three: Harry (our first) and Charlie (our third), and we've found many differences even between these two. Nevertheless, there are certain traits that seem to have been related particularly to their "high-need" personalities, as I've compared them to other children and to their calmer middle brother, Tom. Perhaps identifying some of these "thrills" along the roller-coaster ride of parenting – and the "seat belts" that have helped us survive – will be helpful to other parents of these thrilling, challenging kids.

1. little need for sleep

The *baby* has little need for sleep, that is; you'll crave it constantly! Perhaps this doesn't sound all that unusual. Every parent experiences the wakeful nights in the first few weeks with a newborn, and every grandparent nods along in remembrance. Nights and days can be mixed up, and the baby needs to be fed frequently. Over time, though, the baby develops a rhythm more in harmony with the family, and particularly with his mother if he's breast-feeding. He eventually sleeps for a long period at night, and probably takes a couple of naps during the day, and everyone breathes a sigh of relief.

The high-need child, on the other hand, may not "get it" for a long time. And once she has settled into a routine, it may not last. Furthermore, she may actively resist sleep in a way that can be incredibly frustrating.

Charlie was the most accomplished non-sleeper I've ever seen. It didn't take long to learn that I needed to have him in our bed at night if I wanted to get any rest at all. Still, there were times when I hoped to do other things while he napped.

I had learned with the older boys not to just plunk a napping baby onto cold sheets but to ease him into things, perhaps by lying down to feed him to sleep and then sneaking away, or by laying him down still wrapped in a blanket. I also knew it was important to wait until he was in a sound sleep before sneaking away. Most babies will willingly surrender to sleep under these circumstances. Not Charlie. When he was just a few weeks old, I watched in amazement as he struggled to rouse himself from this deep sleep. I could see his eyes begin to roll under his still-closed eyelids, then his eyebrows would begin to work up and down as he tried to lift open the lids. He would manage to open them just a slit, then close them, then open them a bit wider, then they'd fall closed again. (If you've ever struggled to stay awake while listening to a boring speaker, you'll recognize this description.)

After a real effort, he'd begin to move his body, look around, and cry. And so would I. It was as if he simply could not sleep without being in physical contact with someone, preferably me. He simply would not surrender to this activity that took him out of my arms, no matter how hard he had to struggle against his own body's desperate need for sleep. Even when it was obvious from his behaviour that he was exhausted, he would struggle against the rest he needed.

Nights were worse, because it felt like some sort of planned torture. Charlie would feed to sleep, I'd drift off (you do learn to sleep while feeding when you have a high-need child; you have to), and right in the middle of my own deep sleep, he'd cry. We just couldn't seem to get our sleep cycles in sync. Then it would be difficult for him to go back to sleep. He'd feed and feed and feed. If his mouth relaxed and he let go, he'd startle awake and reach out again. Soon he'd tire of feeding and cry.

As I grew wearier and wearier, I felt like a robot: feed him, bathe him, change him, feed him, rock him, walk him, feed him, cry. At his first cry, the tears would start to my own eyes. I prayed desperately for God to make him sleep. I remember one overwrought night shaking my fist toward the heavens and pleading, "God! Why are you doing this to me? Why won't you make this baby sleep?!"

Over time, and very gradually, he slept better, even if no more. Though he still woke repeatedly at night, we managed to get our sleep cycles synchronized well enough that I was getting a little rest. I had had one hopeful sign when he was about two months old, when he slept through the night – once. Then he didn't do it again for almost two and a half years. And when he did, he dropped his one daytime nap.

My seat belt: there was only one way to keep my sanity with Charlie, and that was to make sleep one of my highest priorities. He spent much of the night in our bed, where I could doze while he fed. Whenever he slept, I slept. Truly important tasks had to get done while he was awake; I was physically incapable of doing anything but what had to be done.

I can see now that the robot mode was really a blessing. By focusing only on what had to be done next, and not worrying about what would come afterward, I managed to get through one day after another. After enough of those days, things improved a bit, and we survived.

Charlie and I had a confrontation when he was about nine months old. It was time for a nap, and I could tell from his mood that he needed it as badly as I did. Still, he would not lie still on the bed. He'd feed a bit, and then crawl and wiggle around in a desperate attempt to prevent himself from surrendering to sleep. Exhausted, I finally said firmly, "You are going to sleep." I rolled him next to me, clasped him tightly against my chest, and didn't let go. He wiggled. He squirmed. He fussed, and then cried. "No", I said, "we're going to sleep." Again and again he tried, and again and again I simply held him tight and insisted that we were going to sleep, and eventually he gave in.

Years later, I have mixed emotions about what I did. With years of parenting him now behind me, I know how stubborn he is; and he probably needed to learn, even that early, that sometimes there is no alternative to what Mum says. On the other hand, I wish I had found a less authoritarian way to urge him to sleep. I keep this memory in my heart as a reminder that while I may have a certain parenting philosophy, sometimes an individual situation seems to offer no alternative, and following the intuition of the moment may be the best approach.

Hope for a smoother track: once Charlie began sleeping through the night, he continued to do so. We've faced occasional nights with nightmares or illness, when he's found his way back into our bed or onto a z-bed beside it. But for the most part, he was happy sharing a room with Tom and now has a room of his own. When he began kindergarten, we established a bedtime and began reading to him and then turning on some favourite music. He still prefers to fall asleep "on the couch with Mum" but will willingly go to bed at our request. Our biggest complaint now is that he sleeps so soundly that he snores! I'm convinced that our constant proof to him that sleep is a pleasant state, not to be feared, is what eventually led to his good sleep habits.

2. high need for mum

I believe the high-need child's desire to avoid sleep is actually related to his need for an awareness of Mum's presence: "If I go to sleep, how will I know she's here?" All babies want Mum close, but the high-need child comes absolutely unglued if she's not there, preferably touching him.

As a small child, Harry exhibited this need by his inability to play in another room. If I was in the kitchen, so was he. If I went into the other room for a moment, he'd follow or cry.

Charlie's need was even greater, manifesting itself especially strongly at church. Even as a tiny baby, he would cry if left in the church crèche – and not just for a few minutes, as the crèche workers always promised, but throughout my absence.

By the time he was three, he willingly went to Sunday school without us. Once when he was about four, I explained to him that I wanted to attend a concert at a campsite where we were staying. I offered him the option of coming with me, where he would have to sit quietly, or going to the childcare centre, where he could play with other children. He agreed it would be more fun to play, and I carefully explained what to expect and when I'd return.

I enjoyed the concert and afterward went to get Charlie. A haggard worker met me at the door. "Thank goodness", she said. "He's been crying ever since you left!" Two hours! For two hours he had cried non-stop, inconsolable, ignoring everyone's efforts to calm him down and interest him in play.

When he was young but had given up feeding, we fell into the habit of watching TV at night with him sitting between my legs, his back against my chest. I would stroke his hair until he drifted off to sleep, and we would then carry him to his bed. Now that he weighs seventy-five pounds and is old enough to be a "tough guy", he still insists on cuddling up for a while every night. He's too heavy – and far too long – to carry, so we try to make sure he doesn't drift off to sleep. If he does, we have to "walk" him to bed, making sure his half-asleep body doesn't run into walls on the way.

My seat belt: call me a wimp if you like; while he was very young, I kept him with me whenever possible. I wanted my child to learn that he didn't need to cry because I would be there when he really needed me. I didn't want him to learn that crying would do no good because I wouldn't respond. At church, I left him in the crèche when he seemed willing but checked several times during the service to make sure he was still content and took him out if he wasn't. (I found that few crèche workers could be trusted to call me, even if I asked them to, because most felt he should cry it out and learn to stay without me.) I then sat in an anteroom where he could play while I listened to as much of the sermon as possible.

We passed up several opportunities for adult activities where children wouldn't be welcome, and took Charlie with us to others where he wouldn't be a real problem. Soon we were able to leave him for brief periods with an older brother or other relative, and eventually he was happy to go to preschool nursery a few mornings a week, as long as he knew Mum would pick him up right on time. We even managed to get away now and then by leaving him at Granny's for a few days.

Hope for a smoother track: really, is it so awful to have a child who loves Mum and desires to spend time with her? It can seem like a burden for a while, and I remember reading of a mum who said spending a day with her toddlers was like being "nibbled to death by ducks". As the child matures, though, and is willing to give mum some breathing space, the mutual affection that has been built up by all the time spent together is an indescribable treasure.

Charlie is an affectionate child and has a tender heart for me when I'm unhappy or upset. Harry, as an adult, has great respect for me and for my opinions, and I treasure him as a friend as much as I do as a son. As wise people have said, you never hear of someone at the end of their life who wishes they had spent less time with their children.

3. high sucking need

All three of my children, including Tom, who was not a high-need child, needed a great deal of sucking stimulus. I suspect that this need exists in everyone to a greater extent than we realize; it's just that some children are more persistent about having it met than others. I can't help but wonder if all the nail biting, gum chewing, and smoking in our society aren't at least a partial reflection of the intensity of a very normal need that didn't get filled and now rises up when stress hits.

My two older boys both sucked their thumbs – avidly. Harry, my first, actually sucked his thumb the day he was born, but then lost the ability to get it to his mouth for a while. (I assume he sucked it in utero.) It was soon rediscovered, though, and his thumb went into his mouth almost as soon as he had finished feeding.

As a first-time parent, it concerned me, and I tried to get him to take a dummy, but he wasn't interested. He would just push it out with his tongue in favour of his thumb. So I looked around at La Leche League meetings, realized

that lots of babies were sucking their thumbs even though they were being breast-fed, and I relaxed. It seemed to me that anything done by so many breast-fed babies using a piece of equipment God had given each of them couldn't be so terrible.

Charlie's sucking need was perhaps no more intense than that of his brothers, but he failed to recognize the value of his thumbs. Instead, he wanted to satisfy his sucking need with me. I found myself wishing Charlie would suck his thumb. I even tried putting it in his mouth! No deal. The dummy didn't interest him either; he wanted to feed – a lot. After a while I gave up, and I used the extensive feeding as an excuse to lie down and rest myself.

Unfortunately, all of this satisfaction of their sucking needs was evidently still not enough. My two high-need children both bite their nails, but then, so did I – until I was out of secondary school (I was also a high-need child). I learned an interesting thing a few years ago, when I met my brothers and sisters from the family that had given me up for adoption. They all bit their nails for years too! This was just one more confirmation for me that the sucking need is natural and intense, and perhaps even more so in a high-need child.

My seat belt: breast-feeding was extremely useful. Aside from the many other advantages, the breast-fed baby must suck harder and longer to satisfy her hunger, so her sucking need gets met as she feeds. Still, some children seem to need even more.

Before having high-need children, I never would have believed I would give this advice:

don't worry about the thumb as long as it's being used to meet an extensive sucking need, and not as a substitute for a parent's presence. You may have to work with the child later to get her to give it up, but she'll be older, and you will be able to use coaxing, reason, and reward.

Hope for a smoother track: children will quit – really. Both of our thumb suckers gave up the habit with a little persuasion. The nail biting has been a bit harder to overcome, but then, to be really honest, I still bite my nails if I'm under a lot of pressure. Again, though, as I look around at all the oral fixations in our culture, I realize how intense this need is. We might as well relax about it a bit with our babies!

4. hyper-responsive to stimuli

Harry and Charlie both showed another common trait among high-need children: the inability to "tune out" stimuli around them. I believe this may have contributed to their difficulty in sleeping.

Most babies and children are able to ignore much of what's going on in their surroundings. There may be twenty other children in a nursery, but many two-year-olds are able to focus intently on the blocks they're playing with and play calmly for a while unless disturbed.

Harry and Charlie weren't able to do this very well. The higher the stimulus level, the higher their activity level would climb. It was

very difficult for them to be calm when more people than just their father and I were around. It was especially hard for Charlie, who had two rowdy brothers to supply constant "electricity".

My worst memory in this regard was a visit from my aunt and uncle when Harry was just two. They were in their sixties and had never had children. They were not very tolerant of children and had strong ideas about how children are supposed to behave.

We had been anticipating the visit, and Harry was responding to the higher-than-usual "charge" in the air with a heightened activity level. My aunt and uncle came in and sat down, and Harry started running through the house for no apparent reason. Before I could catch him to calm him down, he ran up to my aunt, looked her in the eye, and slapped her!

I was appalled and humiliated. I took him into the other room and asked how he could have done such a thing. Still, I could tell that he hadn't intended to be naughty; he was just excited beyond his ability to control himself. There's a difference between wilful misbehaving and a mistake in judgment, and this was clearly the latter. On the other hand, I knew my aunt wouldn't see it that way!

We went back into the family room, and Harry apologized and was quite cooperative after that. Sadly, my aunt never really forgave him. She died when he was a prefect in secondary school, an A student, captain of his football team, and a college scholarship winner, but she was never able to appreciate any of his achievements. She always preferred other nephews. It was her loss.

Charlie has constantly been hyper-responsive to stimuli; it's just plain hard for him to sit still when there's any activity around him. It took a long time for him to learn to sit still through a church service, and we can count on him wanting to leave a restaurant as soon as he's finished, even if the rest of us are still in mid-course. Sometimes we have to impose a five-minute talking moratorium on him during family meals, just to stop his constant, sometimes irrelevant interjections to the conversation. He does much better when just relaxing and watching a TV programme or video (except during commercials, when he's immediately up and bouncing off the walls). There's a noticeable difference when the two of us are alone in the room, as opposed to when Dad and his brothers are watching along with us.

My seat belt: I learned an important lesson from my experiences: a high-need child needs special attention when the stimulus level is high, with excitement in the air for whatever reason. It's wise to "assign" her to a parent (or other familiar person) who can keep an eye out for signs of impending trouble. The child needs help learning to keep her behaviour calm in such circumstances; she also needs parents who insist that she do so while understanding what a struggle it is for her.

Hope for a smoother track: both of our high-need children have mastered this area for the most part. Harry knows himself well enough to seek out the needed quiet to study. On the other hand, if there's fun going on, he's in the middle of

it. That's not a time when he wants to ignore the stimulus!

Charlie has to work on staying calm in school; we've devised a reward system that is helping a great deal. At social events, we still keep an eye on him and try to calm him down when he's getting wound up. He's learning that this is a more difficult problem for him than for other children, and he's trying.

5. hyper when hungry

When Harry was about ten, we took a business/holiday trip to Boston, where the boys and I did some sightseeing. Unfortunately, we had just missed a tour bus and had to kill an hour or so before the next one. We were delighted to find an historic church right next to the terminal and thoroughly enjoyed a tour of it before catching the next bus. However, that meant we were an hour later in finishing the tour than we'd originally planned.

As we walked back to our car, Harry insisted he wanted a bar of chocolate from the corner shop. I refused, saying we'd soon be back at the hotel and would have dinner. He argued, but I held firm. By the time we reached the car, he was irate, insisting that he would not get in the car if I didn't buy him the bar of chocolate. He walked to the other side of the garage and refused to come along. I insisted, but he was equally insistent. If I moved toward him, he dodged and went in another direction. There we were, in a parking lot, in the middle of a strange city, and my child refused to get into the car. I was desperate and I did a foolish thing: I started the car as if to leave, and he relented and came along, but he was in a foul mood all the way back to the hotel.

With this experience, it suddenly dawned on us that many of the times he had been extraordinarily difficult over the years were when he was hungry. With that realization, I remembered that I occasionally become shaky when hungry and feel desperate to eat something quickly, especially if a previous meal or snack was high in sugar. We began to wonder if his unreasonable behaviour was triggered by low blood sugar, and we observed him more closely. It was soon obvious that that was, indeed, the problem. Thankfully, we recognized the same problem early in Charlie.

My seat belt: the obvious solution is to make sure the child doesn't get too hungry. In reality, it's more difficult than that, because circumstances can't always be controlled. If I know we'll be in a situation where we can't control mealtime, I try to take along a snack, such as a cereal bar or small can of fruit juice. Sometimes we've bent our own plans to meet this need, such as by leaving an activity to get something for him to eat, then returning.

Less obvious, but equally important, is to teach the child about his own need. It's impossible to reason with a child in this state, but after the circumstances have passed, we've talked about it. "Charlie", I've explained, "remember this morning when you were really naughty? You were hungry, weren't you? It's really important that you eat when you start to feel that way, so you won't get into trouble again." In this way, he knows I understand how uncontrollable he feels, while realizing that I have to insist on good behaviour, even if he doesn't feel well. I'm also discerning enough to know that all bad behaviour is not due to hunger.

Hope for a smoother track: I'm not certain whether this physical problem tends to resolve itself, or whether the child/adult learns to anticipate and control it. Harry now knows he can be grouchy when he's hungry, so he eats. He's also learned he has to control his temper, and he does – almost all the time. Charlie is still learning; once he's in a difficult state, it's usually up to us to insist he eat something.

6. highly creative

This doesn't seem like a tough one, does it? We all want creative children – or so we think. In reality, we seldom stop to think what that really means.

In our culture, "good" children are ones who do what they're told, without discussion. They sit quietly in their high chairs and eat what they're fed. They obey the Sunday school teacher and take their seat when asked. They don't talk in class at school and they certainly don't argue with their parents.

I've met very few children like that, yet we persist in the fiction. Let me redefine it: many children will do all of these things sometimes; at other times they won't, and their parents or teachers have to insist. A high-need child feels she has to know why she must do them, because she is creative enough to see many other options. Our dear friends Richard and Charlotte Brown, also blessed with two high-need children, had problems with their daughter, Ashleigh, in preschool. It seems she was refusing to complete her work sheets, and the teacher had decided she was a problem child. When her parents asked her why she wouldn't cooperate, she said, candidly, "It's stupid. I already know how to do everything on that paper, so why should I have to do it over and over? I want to learn something new."

And therein lies the dilemma often faced by the parent of a high-need child. We recognize that they must learn to get along in society; they must learn to conform their behaviour to a certain extent. At the same time, we don't want to stifle their inherent creativity and abilities. Where do we draw the line?

My seat belt: I discovered that my perception of a behaviour may need to change. When Harry sat in his high chair and intentionally dropped his cup on the floor the first time, I picked it up and put it back without thought. The second time, it was a little annoying. The third, fourth, fifth time, it got downright frustrating. Then I realized something: I knew it would drop to the floor each time he let it go, but he didn't know that! He was learning about gravity. My job as a parent was to recognize that his behaviour was really understandable, even as I worked to teach him he mustn't drop the cup. Eventually, he stopped – whether because he'd learned the behaviour wasn't acceptable, or because the result was boringly consistent, I don't know. In this case, Harry didn't change. Instead, I learned to value his inquisitiveness.

Hope for a smoother track: if you as a parent can encourage your child to express his creativity in appropriate ways, the rewards can be tremendous. I've been thrilled to watch Harry develop an interest in his schoolwork that has now blossomed into a genuine curiosity about life and a love of learning. Charlie, too, is interested in a variety of things and loves to read.

Friends whose children's creativity tends to be more artistic tell me schoolwork can be a struggle. They seem to have found the greatest success by seeking out alternative methods of learning that take advantage of those abilities, such as special programmes or even home-schooling. And we all benefit when an artistic child learns to channel her creativity into producing things of beauty.

7. resisting authority

Charlie has been particularly insistent at challenging my authority as his mother. In the past my husband's job has required him to travel a great deal. This has meant numerous one- and two-week stretches where I've parented alone, and a major adjustment when he's returned to the family. I might have run into some rough spots while Harry and Tom were young, but Dad was available by phone every evening, and we could usually talk things out. If need be, he spoke to them by phone and reminded them of their responsibilities.

Charlie has been a different story. It's as if he believes that as soon as Dad leaves town, I become vulnerable. He will argue with me incessantly, challenge my authority, refuse to obey me, and even use the emotional weapon every parent dreads: "I don't love you; I hate you. You're mean." His sheer persistence can completely wear me out. Even though I may be firm with him at every point along the way, insisting that he obey, he will come back for more. After a while, I feel as if someone has sucked all the energy out of my body, leaving me just a collapsed shell.

My seat belt: whenever my husband is home, we do "tag-team parenting". One parent takes over for a while when the other gets worn out. Charlie, on the other hand, has needed the "two-parent press", with both of us available nearly all the time to, well, "gang up on him". He has needed to see, quite clearly, that when one parent (usually Mum) was tiring out, the other would take over. And fortunately, my husband does travel less now.

As for school, I've paid careful attention to my children's teachers, even requesting particular ones I felt would understand my children's unique needs. I've done my best to communicate their personalities to their teachers, while offering assurance that we would support the teachers' authority. At the same time, I've worked carefully with the children to help them understand that they must honour authority even when they disagree and use appropriate means to question it without being disrespectful. In an extreme situation, I would not hesitate to request my child be moved to a different classroom. I say that authoritatively, because I learned the hard way – by not making such a request when I should have.

What helps me is to look ahead to the traits I want my child to have as an adult. Do I want him to be a robot, who automatically follows the leader without ever questioning why? Of course not! So I can't stifle his desire to question while he is a child. But neither do I want him to be an arrogant, disrespectful adult who doesn't know how to submit to proper authority. So I must teach him that, too.

A wise, experienced parent, while giving a lecture, was once asked why very bright children can be so difficult. His response applies as well to high-need children (many of whom are gifted as well). My paraphrased recollection of his response is, "A really bright child is very good at almost everything she does. She's very good at maths. She's very good at reading. She's very good at her music lessons. She's very good at arguing with her parents, at getting angry, at being happy or sad."

That answer helped me a great deal to understand my high-need children. Such a child truly can see more of the picture than the average child can, so it's much more difficult for him to yield. As the parent, I believe I must be humble enough to learn from my child when he sees something I don't or haven't thought about. I may be wrong, and I should be big enough to admit it. At the same time, I must be confident enough to trust my own judgment when the child can't see the whole picture. And bright as he may be, his lack of experience will cause him to miss parts of the whole.

Hope for a smoother track: *if* the child learns to respect proper authority, she can work for needed change through appropriate channels. The young people and adults who have learned to harness this energy properly can be a tremendous boon to society. They are our leaders, the ones who have a vision for a better world and who know how to inspire others to participate!

8. stubborn

This conviction on the part of a high-need child that she knows as well – or better – than the adults around her can lead to an astonishing level of stubbornness. With Charlie, it was most apparent in his willingness to undergo a disciplinary action again, and again, and again, and still not give in.

On one occasion I told him he could not go out to play with his friends until he had cleaned his room. Rather than give in, he decided he would simply stay in the room alone. Every so often, I went in with a positive attitude to encourage him to tackle the job, but he was completely unbending. He cried, he yelled, he made a bigger mess than he'd started with – but he would not clean the room. He spent hours in there alone before falling asleep in exhaustion. Eventually he surrendered and cleaned it up, but he'd lost nearly a full day of playing with his friends.

He is also remarkably good at insisting that I fulfil all promises. When he wanted to change the treadmill in his hamster's cage one evening, I felt too weary to tackle another project and promised I would help him do it the next day. When I assessed the situation the next day, I realized it would be a more extensive undertaking than I had anticipated – the cage would have to be completely dismantled and put back together. I tried to talk him out of making the change. "But you promised!" he stubbornly insisted. Who can disagree with the moral imperative of keeping a promise?

It is astonishing which issues Charlie chooses to fight for. They're often not things that are important to every child, such as bedtime or watching a favourite television programme, but rather small issues. I remember Charlie insisting he couldn't drink his orange juice from a glass I had given him, but only from another one. Rather than accept my explanation that the preferred glass was dirty, he demanded "his" glass to the point that I wound up punishing him, and he accepted punishment over and over before finally surrendering. (I wonder now why I didn't simply tell him he could wash the dirty glass if he wanted it so badly.)

Recently, Charlie became so irate about having to leave a baseball team party that he insisted he'd never play again (obviously thinking that would punish us somehow). When I assured him he'd feel differently later, he said, "I won't either. I'm going to cut up my uniform." When he got home, he evidently felt he'd committed himself, so he followed through on his threat by making a snip in his shirt and each sock. I didn't stop him, and he soon felt foolish and submitted to a cooling-off period in his room. He knows better than to complain about the holes he must now wear in his uniform.

My seat belt: to quote Winston Churchill's famous (and short) commencement address, "Never give in, never give in, never, never, never, never – in nothing, great or small, large or petty – never give in except to convictions of honour and good sense." If I decide I'm wrong, of course I back down and admit it. But to surrender to sheer stubbornness on the part of my high-need child would be deadly, because he would only be more stubborn the next time.

Sometimes, as with the baseball uniform, I will allow him to make a mistake and then live with the consequences – a valuable learning tool. But once I've taken a stand, I must hold firm. Full stop.

Hope for a smoother track: can there really be a positive side to this one? Yes! You want an adult who doesn't give up, don't you? Charlie isn't quite there yet, but Harry's dedication made him captain of his football team. His nickname was "Papa", because he was the one who reminded all the other players to keep their heads in the game and follow the rules. He also garnered a prestigious scholarship to college because he didn't give up.

9. negative

A high-need child can have a one-track mind, and that track is often negative. If she decides something is bad, she can focus on it to the exclusion of everything else. The saying "Don't confuse me with the facts, my mind is made up" clearly applies here.

We have found an inexpensive restaurant that the whole family loves. The first time we ate there, we all agreed it was a real find: good food, a fun environment, and cheap. Charlie really liked his meal. One day not long after, we decided to return to our discovery. Charlie wanted to go somewhere else, so he informed us that he hated the restaurant we had chosen. We reminded him of what he had eaten and how much he liked it. "No, I didn't. It was terrible", he replied. We mentioned the things we'd enjoyed about the atmosphere, and he insisted he had hated that too. We made it clear, "That's where we're going; there's no use arguing about it." All the way to the restaurant, he pouted in the corner of the car. He pouted while we ordered. Of course, as soon as he got his food, he devoured it, and even commented how good it was. Just two weeks after that, we decided again to go back to our favourite, and what was his reaction? "I hate that place."

Charlie is one of those people who insist on seeing the dark side of the situation, instead of the light, even to the point of being completely unwilling to see reality. If he decides it's time to go to baseball practice and I'm not quite ready, he says, "We're going to be a half hour late." If I ask him to wait a moment before he changes the television channel, he complains, "I'm going to miss the whole show!" If the teacher has sent a paper home Monday to be returned by the end of the week, it has to go back Tuesday, "or I'll really get in trouble".

Charlie loves doing schoolwork papers, but once in a while he runs into one he doesn't immediately "get". Before I can complete even a sentence of explanation, he storms from the room, crying, "I can't do it." Sometimes we can tackle it again later, when he's calm, but there have been a few times I've had to either insist he complete an important paper or allow him to leave the work undone and ask the teacher for assistance the next day.

My seat belt: this child needs a great deal of help seeing what's good about life, even when he can't have his own way. It's one of the more difficult challenges the parent of a high-need child faces, and the only suggestion I have is be positive yourself, and hang in there.

Hope for a smoother track: hopefully, the negative outlook will pass as the child's experiences teach him that things are often better than they may seem at first. Charlie actually seemed happy last time we went to our restaurant. He still gets anxious about getting schoolwork done ahead of time, but that's not really such a big problem, is it?

This trait can be a positive one in adults, if they can couple their tendency to notice what needs to be improved with a drive for positive change. It helps if they have friends and co-workers who remind them to lighten up.

10. opinionated

Both of my high-need children have been terrific arguers. They can often come up with better arguments to change my decision than I can muster to stick to it. And they are absolutely convinced they're right.

On a recent motorway ride after shopping, Charlie asked if we could ride "up on the ramp" he said paralleled the motorway. Neither his dad nor I could figure out what he meant, so he offered a further description. Since we are both very familiar with that stretch, we explained that there was no ramp we could take, but only those that are entrances or exits, including some connections to another motorway going in a different direction. Charlie insisted. His father patiently explained that he drives that road frequently and that Charlie misunderstood the purpose of the ramp. Still he persisted. We were wrong, and he could show us!

In exasperation, Dad said, "When we get home, we'll drop off Mum and the packages, and I'll drive you back to show you you're wrong. Is that what you want me to do? Or is it just possible this might be one of those times when you could be wrong?" Charlie stopped short of insisting they go back, but he obviously was not convinced.

My seat belt: this is a tough one. In exasperation, we have at times resorted to simply insisting that Charlie is wrong and that we will accept no more argument on a subject. Whenever possible, we've proven his mistake, because we want him to learn that he is not infallible. At the same time, we don't want to humiliate him when he's mistaken.

I've chosen to allow my children to discuss things with me; that's different from arguing. Over time, they are learning to make a clear, concise case for their position.

We've worked to get Charlie to admit that he is occasionally mistaken, and we're trying to teach him to acknowledge that any particular situation could be one of those times. We also explain that there are times when two people simply will not reach agreement – either because one is wrong and doesn't realize it, or because they may have different perspectives, both of which may be right – and that in those times, it's all right to "agree to disagree". With an insistent high-need child, though, this is a difficult task that requires constant repetition. Finally, we've explained that he must yield to our authority, even if he believes we are wrong.

Hope for a smoother track: some high-need children become more reasonable as they mature. However, though Harry has learned to surrender more gracefully when he is wrong, as an adult he is a more formidable opponent than ever when convinced he's right. He and I have stimulating debates on politics, ethics, and other challenging issues – and I lose more often than I'd like! I believe he's going to be a tremendous influence for good wherever he finds himself. What more could a parent want?

11. high need for affirmation

I have to be kidding, right? I've given one example after another of how insistent this child can be. Isn't he overconfident? Well, my high-need children weren't. Each one of them needed an extraordinary amount of support and encouragement.

This didn't always show up right away; they were often willing, even eager, to tackle new things. But if it didn't work out immediately, they lacked confidence to keep trying, and they needed constant support.

Baseball makes this need particularly obvious. Charlie's Little League teammates barely seem to notice their parents in the stands, electing instead to take congratulations or criticism from their fellow players. Not Charlie. Every time he comes out of the dugout, he looks to the stands to be sure we're not only present, but watching. After a couple of practice swings, he looks again. As he walks to the plate, he looks up another time, to make certain he has our attention. At each base where he makes a stop, he looks again and smiles sheepishly. It's vitally important to him to know we're there and that we care.

My seat belt: we point out and celebrate Charlie's victories to boost his confidence for the next challenge. When he feels he just can't do something, past victories may provide support to try again. We encourage him to try new things, "just once". He may find out he likes them, as he did with baseball.

At the same time, we've found it important to insist that he not give up too easily since that undermines his confidence. Before we allowed Charlie to join a Little League team, we made it clear that he was making a commitment to be part of the team, and we would not allow him to quit if he decided he didn't like it, because that would be letting other people down. Sure enough, he got discouraged for a while and wanted to quit, but we didn't give in, and he soon decided he liked it after all and wanted to play the next year. He began this year's season saying he probably wouldn't play next year, when he'd have to face harder pitchers, but before the season was over, his own batting success and improved fielding had him saying he would stick with it next year too.

If a child who needs affirmation really was not doing well at something, and it was undermining her confidence rather than boosting it, I would allow her to quit rather than face real discouragement – but I would balance that with another activity at which I thought she could succeed as soon as possible.

Hope for a smoother track: experience, experience, experience. Each time Charlie succeeds at something, it puts fuel in his "confidence tank." Baseball success emboldened him to try karate. Enjoying karate seems to be encouraging him to try a summer class about the rain forest this year. And he's learned that he got good at these things only by sticking to them, even when he wanted to quit.

As a parent, I've found it very rewarding to encourage my child (sometimes insist) to persevere, and then to see his face light up when he gets a trophy. It's a struggle sometimes not to brag about my sons' achievements in school and activities. Please forgive me – I'm a proud parent!

12. "it's not my fault!"

Another challenge we've faced consistently with both our high-need children, but particularly with Charlie, has been their difficulty accepting responsibility for their actions. Their creativity aids them in finding reasons others are at fault. Their stubbornness may be the reason it's so difficult for them to accept their own responsibility.

Charlie has had some struggles getting along with other children his own age, largely because he wants to be in charge, and the others don't always want to follow his suggestions. Whenever he comes home after a battle with one of his friends, I can expect to hear a full, minutely detailed explanation of why it was so-and-so's fault, not his. Sometimes he gets extremely angry.

We've had the same difficulty at school, where he is obedient but has a very hard time staying quiet in class. The explanation is always, "Adam talked to me; I was only telling him to be quiet", or, "It was my turn and he wouldn't let me, so I had to talk."

My seat belt: I've had to learn to leave Charlie no room to "hide". I press for more and more details until I can get a full picture of what happened. If that doesn't work, I might ask, "If I call Ms C and ask her, what will she say happened?" On occasion I've got both children together after an argument and asked each to tell their story in front of the other. The point: Charlie is learning that while everyone is inclined to present himself or herself in a more favourable light, he will ultimately have to acknowledge what he could have done differently, and that we expect him to act differently the next time.

Hope for a smoother track: I really believe my children's consciences benefit by learning to accept responsibility. Not doing so leaves a nagging feeling inside that they really were wrong, but they got away with it. Charlie's countenance has actually lit up once he's been caught, corrected, and forgiven. The real reward has been when he's confessed wrongdoing that we hadn't discovered, because he wants the clear conscience that comes from owning up. We're still working on it, but I'm thrilled at the signs of his growing maturity.

where do i go to resign?

I hope reading about my experiences hasn't made you feel like giving up. Remember – most of us enjoy roller coasters, if we can surrender to the fun of the ride. The high-need child is exasperating, but she can be extremely rewarding. A child who is very good at being angry or argumentative also can be very good at being loving, at rubbing your back, at comforting a distressed sibling. The dips on the high-need roller coaster may seem very low, but the peaks are thrilling. And having adult children as friends is incredibly rewarding.

So don't resign. Instead, devote yourself to meeting your high-need child's needs, and enjoy the ride!

chapter 12

disciplining the high-need child

Difficult to discipline ranks high on the complaint list of parents with high-need children: "He's so stubborn", "She just won't obey", "He runs wild", "She's so defiant." High-need children are so challenging to discipline because the same temperament traits that make them creative and interesting also get them into trouble.

Intense and curious children have a head start in learning, but these traits can also make them impulsive and exhausting. Persistent, strong-willed personalities have no trouble with confidence and assertiveness, but without discipline these traits can turn into disobedience and defiance. Disciplining the high-need child requires balance. A highly restrictive and negative atmosphere sets up parent and child for endless power struggles and days full of nos, and squelches the positive traits in a child's personality. Yet lazy discipline that sets no limits for children causes them to run wild.

Disciplining children during the infant and toddler stages makes them easier to live with and discipline at later ages. The home is their first social group, a sort of mini-society that prepares them for later life. How the child behaves with his parents teaches him how to behave with other people. Peers, teachers, and employers will be less accepting than you of your high-need child's temperament and are likely to label your child stubborn, bossy, argumentative, and so on. By disciplining your child from infancy onward, you give him the tools to control himself and get along within the family. These skills will carry over into relationships later on, helping your child get along in the world at large.

Discipline is something you do with and for a child, not something you do to a child. Expect discipline to be your greatest challenge with your high-need child; it will also be the source of the greatest rewards. In some ways it is more difficult to discipline a high-need child; in others it is actually easier. Because these children are so intense and supersensitive, they seem to have an innate sense of fairness and justice, so that if they truly understand what behaviour is expected of them and why, they are more likely to comply.

Regardless of your child's need level, one of your parenting goals is to help him acquire self-discipline. Children are searching for a norm, for how they are supposed to behave. The home is a boot camp for training children and giving them the tools to behave in a larger society that is less accepting and less tolerant than their home. If the child sees gentleness yet firmness and structure yet flexibility, and perceives that discipline is part of your love and care for him, he regards this caring, responsive way of life as the norm. He learns it is normal to speak softly rather than yell. It is normal to hug rather than hit. It is normal to meet others' needs. Every interaction the child perceives in normal daily living becomes part of him and his inner guidance system, his self-discipline.

Parents are often confused about discipline, especially when they have a strong-willed child who is resistant to common discipline techniques. Before looking at the "how to" of discipline, it helps to understand the real meaning of the concept.

Disciplining a child, high-need or not, means determining how you need your child to behave in order to like living with your child, conveying this expected behaviour to the child, and then coming up with creative ways to make this happen.

Our family swimming pool is not only a place of recreation, it's a place for relaxation. One day I was swimming with our three- and six-year-old children and they began whining and pestering each other. I got their attention and said, "This is our happy pool. We have only happy sounds in our happy pool." Then I performed a few happy antics to show them the behaviour I expected. The children then knew the pool rules and I again liked swimming with them.

"Discipline" also means teaching and training. It involves:

- Building a close relationship with your child. Your relationship with your child is the cornerstone of effective discipline.
- Liking your child. Children who are genuinely liked will grow up believing they are likable.
- Developing a mutual sensitivity between you and your child. It's important for the parent and child to be able to read each other's moods and needs; if you are able to get behind the eyes of your child, you will be able to understand your child's behaviour from one situation to the next.
- Letting your child know exactly what kind of behaviour you expect. Many children don't know what is acceptable or unacceptable behaviour until you tell them. High-need children, especially, require frequent reminders to reinforce your expectations.
- Helping your child respect your authority, as well as the authority of others.
- Structuring your child's environment to encourage desirable behaviour.
- Modelling self-discipline to your child.
- Helping your child develop inner controls.
- Helping your child develop a sense of responsibility.
- Helping your child make wise choices.
- Developing techniques that encourage desirable behaviour.

Notice that we have listed techniques last. This is because techniques, usually advice from "experts", are often no more than quick-fix gimmicks that sound good in books and lectures but may not work with your child. Disciplining a high-need child involves more than simply hitting on the right bunch of techniques. These children are notoriously resistant to tricks and methods, especially when they involve corporal forms of punishment. They see right through them. With a high-need child, you must work on building a genuine discipline relationship. With this foundation you may not have to rely on the discipline gimmick of the week.

get connected to your child – early

The stronger your parent-child connection, the easier it will be to discipline your child. You may not have considered the many hours of holding your baby, the seemingly constant feeding, the repeated nurturing response to your baby's cries, day and night, as acts of discipline, but they were. The more hours per day a parent and child are in touch with each other and interact with each other, the better they get to know each other. The high-touch style of attachment parenting lays the foundation of discipline: knowing your child. When you know your child well, you know what conditions encourage desirable behaviour and what situations are a set-up for misbehaviour. Forming a deep connection with your child helps you anticipate

and take action before your child has a chance to get into serious trouble. You tailor your discipline to the child's needs rather than persisting with a technique that is not working.

Not only are connected parents able to read their child well, but connected children are also better able to read their parents. Connected kids more easily know what behaviour their parents expect. They also understand their parents' moods and become sensitive to their parents' body language. Because of this mutual sensitivity, these children naturally want to please their parents. Connected kids are set up to obey.

Getting connected to your infant by practising the high-touch style of attachment parenting we described in Chapter 1 is the best

excuses, excuses

Labelling children high-need is a mixed blessing. On the one hand, it explains their behaviour and the kind of parenting they need. Yet it is easy for even the wisest parent to fall into the trap of lax discipline because of this label. The term "high-need" explains a child's behaviour, but it doesn't excuse it. Yes, you will need to widen your acceptance of what is "normal" behaviour to mean what is normal for your child, but don't let yourself hide behind this label to the extent that your child runs wild. If your child is being obnoxious and disrupting the whole playgroup, it's time to intervene. "High-need" doesn't mean your child is allowed to misbehave. It simply means he needs a more creative style of discipline.

preventive discipline "technique" for any child, especially a high-need child. If you are having problems with your child, take a look at your relationship with your child before trying a bunch of techniques. If you have had a distant relationship with your child since infancy and your connection is still a bit shaky, work first on strengthening the relationship. You will find that discipline will naturally become easier.

How do you get reconnected? Spend more time with your child. Try to see the world through her eyes. Do things with your child and have fun together. This is especially helpful if your child is in a negative phase and your days have been full of nos. Several parents from my practice have successfully turned around their relationship with their high-need children simply by spending more time with them. One mother home-schooled her six-year-old for a year. A father took his four-year-old with him on frequent business trips. The child felt so special that her negative attitude turned positive. Frequent opportunities for connecting can overcome a child's resistance to her parents' discipline.

It is never too late to begin to practise attachment parenting. Children are resilient. They are able to bounce back from a difficult start. They seldom carry grudges and memories of one bad day into the next. Yet one of the reasons we stress the importance of attachment parenting from birth is that the earlier you get connected to your child, the easier discipline – and everything else – will be. Deep connections are not built in a day, nor are children's attitudes changed overnight. It may take many months to reconnect with your child and form a deep attachment that will make discipline more effective for you. One mother of a high-need child realized that the root of her discipline problem was a distant relationship between her and her child. She vowed to keep working at the relationship until they both felt connected. She described this process: "It was like camping out with our five-year-old for a year." Shorten the distance between yourself and your child; you will find discipline to be much easier at this close range.

There really are some wonderful rewards for putting all that time and energy into parenting a difficult baby. A good example in our case is the subject of discipline. One would expect Ellie to be difficult to discipline, but I have not found that to be true. Perhaps because we have had such a close, intimate relationship, she really listens to me. I know her inside and out, and I can usually tell what she is thinking. This makes certain discipline techniques, such as verbal instruction, explanation of logical consequences, and modelling (the best of all) very effective tools in teaching her about the world and her place in it.

study your child

You must become the expert on your high-need child; no one else will be able to understand your child as well as you will. The three key words for disciplining a high-need child at any age are *know your child*. Along with knowing your individual child, it helps to know age-appropriate behaviour: what is usual and

for better or for worse ...

A high-need child can be an asset or a liability. Depending on your attitude, living with a high-need child can become an opportunity for growth, a chance to hone your parenting skills, sharpen your sensitivity, and even smooth some rough edges in your own personality. Or, it can be a negative experience, one filled with frustration as you struggle to make your child into the child you wish you had instead of valuing the person she really is. One of the most frequent statements we hear from parents of high-need children is, "This experience has made me a better parent, and a better person." Your child's personality is not within your control, but whether your experience is generally positive or negative is up to you.

normal behaviour for most children at various stages of development.* Discovering that most two-year-olds love to say no and learning about why this is so will make it easier to cope with your own little nay-sayer. Knowing your child and his developmental stage will help you keep your behavioural expectations in line with his capabilities.

---

* For guidelines to understanding age-appropriate behaviour, see *The Discipline Book*, by William Sears and Martha Sears (Thorsons, 2005).

think kid first

Disciplining a high-need child calls for a change in mind-set. You have to learn to think first from your child's perspective. Children often do irritating things, but instead of reacting with adult thoughts such as "How inconvenient for me" or "He's challenging my authority", get inside your child's mind. Try to see his viewpoint, why he is doing what he is doing.

Lauren, who is now three and a half, has been in her independent mode for quite a while. We have learned how to allow this to unfold and develop without letting it undermine our authority. By our understanding Lauren's point of view and not allowing ourselves to get drawn into angry confrontations, we have been able to weather this lengthy declaration of independence. For example, the other evening we had a cheer squad sleepover, which involved just about everything but sleep. Lauren was enjoying herself immensely. When Martha announced story time at 9pm, Lauren politely but emphatically let her know that she'd just stay up with the big girls and Martha could go to bed by herself. Martha sat down with her to listen to her plans while she held a mental dialogue with herself concerning her options. As Lauren talked, Martha reaffirmed in her own mind that "stories followed by bed" was the only way to go in light of her own reserves and level of tiredness. As she listened, she was giving Lauren a look that let her know that her plans were not an option. She didn't argue or use force (this always backfires with Lauren). After a few minutes of calmly listening, without one shred of encouragement that Lauren's plans might work, Martha held out her hand and said, "Come on with me, Lauren, and we'll pick out some stories." She took Martha's hand (feeling that she still had some choice in the matter) and trotted off to our bedroom with her.

You will find that discipline will work much better for you once you consider your child's viewpoint in your disciplinary actions. This does not mean that you are losing your authority or letting your child dictate the discipline; it simply means that you respect your child's viewpoint too. Parents who feel they have to be in constant control may have difficulty switching into "kid first" mode. Once you overcome your need to feel in control and realize that considering your child's needs in your decision making is actually part of being in charge, you will find your relationship with your child much smoother. Having to have it your way, no matter what, sets you up for days full of negative interactions. (This does not imply martyr-mothering. Often you have to think, "Mum first". What's good for mother is ultimately good for the child.)

provide structure, set limits

"Structure" here means conditions that encourage your child to behave. You become like an environmental engineer, structuring your child's day, his play activities, his homework, his schooling, whatever it takes to help your child succeed and behave. Structuring your child's environment requires that you have mastered the first three building blocks of discipline: being connected to your child, knowing your child, and being able to walk in your child's shoes. To structure your child's environment, you put all this information together and use it to keep a few steps ahead of your child. For example, high-need children are notoriously impatient. They have difficulty waiting in lines in restaurants or waiting their turn in games. Ignoring this trait sets your child up for trouble. Instead, structure the situation by choosing a restaurant or time to dine where there will be no lines, and choose games that require a minimum amount of waiting. (We found out the hard way that six-year-old Stephen did much better playing soccer than he did baseball because he needed to be running with the pack. He did not need to be sitting in the outfield playing in the dirt while he waited for his turn at bat.)

fitting in

Regardless of temperament or level of need, every child needs to learn to fit into the family environment and observe house rules. Adaptability is necessary in life. Later on, children will have to adapt themselves to many different social settings. Learning adaptability begins at home. While it is true that parents must increase their acceptance of childlike behaviour from high-need children, they must discipline behaviour that hurts others, hurts property, or is just downright obnoxious. We have found it helpful to divide our children's undesirable behaviours into biggies and smallies. We waste little energy on smallies and concentrate on fixing the biggies.

Because of their strong persistence, high-need children challenge limits. Yet setting limits is a necessary part of disciplining any child, especially a high-need child. Structure makes limit-setting easier. For example, you establish house rules, what the child may and may not touch. High-need children are very curious and explorative and will want very much to touch the things they are not supposed to. Structuring a child's play environment by toddler-proofing your home makes obeying the house rules easier for your child. You simply remove as many of the no-touches as you can and let your curious child enjoy a fascinating array of yes-touches. Structure is not confining. It is just the opposite; it means you're setting up your child's environment to encourage desirable behaviour. By using your adult creativity to provide a framework within which your child can comfortably and safely play, you free your child to become a curious explorer. All children need limits and boundaries, but for high-need children these may need to be defined more creatively. For some children, placing the DVD out of reach may be enough. For high-need children, it may need to go under lock and key, or you may have to teach them how to use it carefully at an early age.

Plan ahead. Providing structure also implies anticipating disciplinary problems and situations that set your child up for undesirable behaviour. Thinking ahead, you programme your child's day to encourage desirable behaviour. You know when your child is likely to be in a good mood and the times of the day and situations that bring out the worst behaviour.

Therefore, you plan your shopping trips for the good-mood times and be sure your child is well rested and well fed before outings. You choose playmates, play situations, and times for group play that you have learned work best.

Set routines. Most high-need children thrive on routines. They need to know what to expect. For example, a set bedtime routine of quiet time, brush teeth, bedtime story, back rub, song, and so on, will help these children settle down to sleep. There is comfort in familiar routines for bedtime, mealtimes, or for getting ready to go out.

know when to say yes and when to say no

Remember, disciplining the high-need child requires striking a balance. Discipline calls for a balance between saying yes and saying no and having the wisdom to know when to say which. Because of their persistence and their natural preoccupation with their own agenda, high-need children are often unfairly labelled "stubborn" and "defiant". It is easy to fall into the trap of overreacting to these traits, coming down too hard on the child, saying and then yelling no all day long. This will turn the potentially positive trait of persistence into sullen defiance and will create distance between parent and child. The other extreme – avoiding saying no at all costs – allows the child to control the household and run wild. This child will have little or no self-control as an adult.

Realize that you must set limits. There are times when you, practically speaking, must say no. Otherwise, you will drive yourself crazy, and your child will never learn to deal with frustration. Saying no may be especially difficult for parents who have practised the high-touch style of attachment parenting in the first two years. Especially in the first year, you were almost totally a "yes" parent as you fed your child on cue and responded to your child's cries. However, needs change as a baby grows into a toddler and preschooler. Saying yes to your growing child's need for limits will often involve saying no to your child's impulsive behaviour. The foundation of trust you laid during infancy will make this easier.

Dealing with a high-need child literally is a process of making deals. Negotiating and dealing may offend the authority figure in parents who feel they have to be in control. Yet this is not a weakness but simply a matter of survival. Persistent kids often have difficulty saying no to themselves and actually need someone to say no for them. It's a relief to persistent kids to know they don't have so much power to derail their parents. Negotiating with children is not the same as negotiating in the United Nations; parent and child do not have equal votes. High-need children need the security of having an authority figure in charge, though they may not always realize it, and many have difficulty accepting authority figures. The earlier you teach them how to work with authority figures, the smoother their lives will be. Throughout their lives they will encounter many authority figures in school and at work. The tools you give them now will make it easier for them to accept and work with authority figures who may not be so understanding or compromising.

Living with my three-year-old, Andrew became much easier once I learned to make "deals" that worked to my advantage, yet didn't threaten my authority. Sometimes instead of going to bed, he wants to watch a video. I say, "Okay, we'll make a deal. Get in your pyjamas, brush your teeth, go to the potty, and we'll watch a video together." Ten minutes into the video he's asleep.

Persistent children see only their viewpoint. If you rush in to say no to their demand too quickly, you set yourself up for an unfruitful power struggle. Here are creative ways to say no, yet at the same time create a positive attitude in your very positive little person.

Listen to the child's viewpoint. Nothing wins over a high-need child like respect for her needs. Be sympathetic as you talk with her and encourage her to explain her need. Many times a child allowed to vent her feelings will literally talk herself out of her perceived need. Ten-year-old Erin insisted on seeing a movie that we didn't approve of. Persistently she pleaded her case; it seemed to her that her life simply couldn't go on unless she saw this movie. We let her state her case without interruption, offering an occasional, sympathetic phrase to show her we understood how difficult it is to want something your parents refuse to let you have: "You really want to see that movie, don't you?" "A lot of your friends will see it." "Tell me what's so special about this movie." "You really would feel cheated if you missed that movie."

handling car seat protests

While car rides soothe many fussy babies, high-need infants often protest being confined in a car seat. Try these travel tips if your baby goes berserk on car rides: for younger babies, consider limiting car trips as much as possible. Keep the trips short, under ten minutes. If you need to go a longer distance, consider having someone else drive you so you'll be free to concentrate on baby, even feed as you ride along. Martha found that our babies came to understand that if I was driving, she could feed them; they'd cry more when they realized she was driving. (Eventually, as they grew older, they also realized that when Martha was driving they'd have to be content with verbal and visual contact – they figured out that when she was in the driver's seat she wouldn't be able to feed them.)

Feed your baby without removing him from the car seat. This way the driver doesn't have to stop, and baby won't be disturbed. Sit next to your infant and keep your seat belt buckled while you lean in toward the car seat. You may end up with a few stiff muscles, but the peace and quiet may be well worth it. One day I was driving our van while Martha was sitting behind me with ten-month-old Erin, who was crying inconsolably, in her toddler car seat. As I looked into the rear view mirror, I saw a breast meet Erin's eager mouth. Erin's cry stopped instantly and she soon drifted off to sleep. It was such a strange thing to see in

the mirror that I nearly ran off the road, but the rest of the trip was peaceful. Martha and I had a good laugh over our first "exposure" to using the breast to comfort a car-seated baby.

Safety comes before psychology. It's important that your baby learn that being in a car seat is a nonnegotiable fact of family life. We learned the hard way to never, ever take a baby out of the car seat. When Erin was only three weeks old, we had an accident on the motorway just ten minutes after Martha had put Erin back into her seat after having taken her out to calm her by feeding.

Whenever possible, time your travel during baby's best moods. Leave a bag of toys in your car that are reserved only for travel time. Offer your child one interesting toy during each trip. Play favourite tapes that are reserved just for car time. As baby gets older you can offer non-chokable, non-messy finger foods to keep him satisfied. Although our babies weren't fed from bottles, we did try using a water bottle once they were old enough to manage it on their own in their car seat. It worked for one or two of them.

Timothy hated his car seat. Rather than falling asleep in the car as many infants do, he would work his way up to screaming and would continue to scream the whole time I was driving. Needless to say, it was unnerving. I realized that if I stayed peaceful through the ride he would settle down. When I became angry with him and upset about his screams, I noticed it would take a longer time to calm him down when the ride was over. So I learned to sing songs during the ride and stay peaceful. He eventually caught the happy spirit of the car ride.

One day, when we accidentally turned the radio on loud, Stephen, who at six months was crying a lot in the car, suddenly stopped. It happened to be inspirational music of the type he heard a lot in our home and at church. Hearing it in the car probably gave him a sense of being connected to the familiarity of home and good feelings. He quieted instantly whenever he heard it, and he heard it a lot from then on! For Stephen, having it loud was part of the discovery – he liked the extra stimulation. Other babies may be disturbed by the loudness; you'll have to experiment. Choose music you like too, since you will have to hear it a lot. There are many delightful children's tapes available. Rotate them for variety.

Hayden was such a basket case in her car seat that Martha was inspired to make up two songs that she sang to Hayden (and all subsequent children) to make her laugh. The first can be sung to the tune of the ABC song:

> *Seat belt, seat belt, seat belt off!*
> *Seat belt, seat belt, off off off!*
> *Take my seat belt off right now.*
> *Or I'll scream and throw a cow*
> *(in the swimming pool*
> *[added in a monotone as an aside])*
> *Seat belt, seat belt, seat belt off!*
> *Seat belt, seat belt, off off off!*

For this song, make up your own tune (Martha's tune is an original):

> *I don't like my car seat.*
> *I don't like my car seat.*
> *It makes me sit*
> *It makes me be*
> *As quiet*
> *As a mousie.*

The more Erin talked, the more she saw the weakness of her arguments; she realized that her life could go on even if she missed the movie. High-need children are not wimpy kids. Only after we showed enough respect for Erin's viewpoint to listen and sympathize could she open herself to our viewpoint. We presented our side of the discussion, why we believed the movie was not good for her.

Finally, we offered an alternative we knew that she would accept.

In order to discipline the high-need child you must become a good listener. Years of doing this will allow you to see the payoff when your child is older. Nothing wins over a high-need teenager like the feeling that his parents truly understand his viewpoint – whether or not they agree with it.

Give positive substitutes. After saying no, quickly interject an acceptable alternative before your child has a chance to protest: "You may not have the sharp knife, but you may help me mash the potatoes" (or scrub the sink, or slice apples with this table knife, or help tear the lettuce for the salad …). Offering an attractive substitute catches your child by surprise and preserves his sense of curiosity and adventure.

When my two older girls were young, I would tell them not to touch certain things and they would obey. With Amy, we can see a real need to touch that favourite, breakable heirloom. No matter how many times we pull her away, she will go right back and stand looking at it, inching her finger ever so close. But if we let her hold it for a few moments and tell her it belongs to mummy, she will be satisfied and not touch it again.

Choose alternatives to "no". High-need children quickly learn the power of the word "no". If they hear it too often from you, they will turn it against you and say no to all of your requests. Use words like "hurt", "dirty", "yuck", or "stop". Save "no" for the big issues, and your child won't be deaf to the word when you really need to get your point across. This doesn't mean that you have to completely eliminate the N word from your child-discipline vocabulary. Over the past several years, I have noticed a sort of pseudo-positive discipline style creeping into popular books and magazine articles that advises parents to "keep the child's atmosphere positive and never use negatives". Some day nurseries even have rules forbidding the nannies to use any negative explanation when disciplining the children. This is unrealistic. The world is full of yeses and nos. All children, especially high-need ones, need to learn how to accept no when important issues are involved.

A friend of ours, a mother of five and a wise disciplinarian who was working with two-year-olds in a day care, was seriously reprimanded for calling out sharply to a child across the room who was about to bite his playmate, "No biting!" Her quick action actually saved the other child from being bitten, yet she was required by her supervisor to go to a series of classes to learn "positive discipline". While positive discipline is important, it's often had disastrous results, especially in an educational system where teachers spend more time disciplining than teaching. Trying to rephrase a simple "no" directive in a nice-sounding positive "teeth are for eating" instead of "don't bite" comes out as strained and unnatural, and has a non-serious ring. Besides, children often perceive these wimpy positives as phoney.

Personalize the negative. A phrase we have successfully used for our two- and three-year-olds is "not for Lauren (Stephen, etc.)." It communicates that there is something special about the child that causes this item to be not for her. Hearing her name tacked onto the "no" seems to soften the blow and encourages the child to redirect her attention to something that is appropriate for her.

Offer a "yes" environment. High-need children need space where they can just be kids. If your day begins with cries of "no" and "don't touch" and deteriorates into whines and tantrums, you need a positive change of scenery. Parks and playgrounds provide a "yes" environment. Go to a friend's house. Children's activity centres, full of yes-touches, are springing up in many towns and cities. These are indoor playgrounds, many in shopping centres, where a parent can sit and relax while children are free to roam, put their hands on everything, and explore in a safe and interesting environment without getting lost.

command respect

Don't "lose it" and reduce yourself to your child's level. Remain the secure, trustworthy adult who is in charge. Angry rages frighten the sensitive child, disgust the discerning child, or encourage the impish child to try harder to get mum or dad to "blow their top". With any of the above, you are no longer in the position of leadership. Leaders command respect by giving respect. When you throw your own tantrum, you are not respecting either your child or yourself. How then can you expect him to respect you? Those of us who have trouble staying calm and peaceful in the face of irritation (and we all do, some much more than others) will find this area of parenting much more doable once we figure out how to control our own inner alarms. (See Chapter 7, "Mother Burnout".)

help your child learn empathy

High-need children are prone to impulsive behaviour. They act before they think. This prevents them from considering the effects of their actions on others. Your parenting can influence whether your child becomes an empathic or an uncaring adult. High-need children are sensitive – they feel deeply, care deeply, and react intensely. They are easily bothered. With your help, this trait can help your child become sensitive to others. When you respond sensitively to your child's needs, thinking "kid first" (as discussed on page 188) and when you try to understand his viewpoint, he learns that this way of communicating and interacting with people is the norm. Your modelling conveys that you expect your child to consider the needs of other people, just as you have considered his needs. This is the beginning of teaching your child empathy.

If, on the other hand, the child becomes accustomed to a more distant, restrained style of parenting, one that ignores his viewpoint, he comes to see this "me first", uncaring style of interaction as the norm. This child is not likely to consider the effects of his behaviour on another person before he acts. His own impulses are valued more highly than the needs of others. Lack of empathy, not feeling remorse, and not considering the effects of what one does are the hallmarks of sociopathic behaviour. As one mother of a high-need child once said to us, "Teaching my child to be a caring person is the best way to later keep him out of jail." (For further discussion on the topic of empathy, see page 218.)

To lead your child to consider how his behaviour will affect another person, try these exercises:

"How would you feel?" Ask your six-year-old to imagine his own feelings if he were on the receiving end of certain behaviour. "How would you feel if Billy grabbed your ball?" "How would you feel if Suzy hit you?" The high-need child's sensitivity will easily lead him to understand the hurtful outcome of these acts. However, most high-need children are prone to act impulsively, so it may take lots of practice before empathy can overcome impulse. Helping your child learn to project his feelings onto others pre-programmes him to consider the effects of his behaviour on others, thinking, "others first" in the same way that his parents learned to think "kid first" (see page 188).

The Golden Rule applies here. Do unto your child as you would have him do unto others. Model how you expect him to treat other people. Grabbing things from your child, yelling at him, and hitting him give the child the message that this is how people treat people.

From the moment Jessica was born I regarded her as a spiritual being, not just a body. I treated her as if she had all the emotions, feelings, and needs of any other person and with as much respect and dignity as any adult. I don't believe in teasing or talking down to a child or making less of them. I assume that Jessica is good and wants to do good. When directing her actions, I act on that and try

to guide her. At two and a half years old, she is not spoiled as people suggested would happen; it's just the opposite. She is affectionate, happy, outgoing, independent, and very sociable. She seems unusually sensitive to the feelings of others. She has been talking in sentences since about eighteen months, counting and reciting rhymes; and we seem to have missed the "terrible twos". She actually wants to cooperate.

Take advantage of "teachable times". Simply spending a lot of time with your child will give you plenty of opportunities to teach empathy. This is valuable anticipatory discipline to prevent children from infringing upon the rights of others. Once I was walking with our son Matthew when we saw a couple of local boys throwing water balloons at cars. This was a teachable moment where I could show Matthew and the other boys the importance of considering how their actions affect others. I sat down with the boys and began the following dialogue:

"You guys certainly like to throw water balloons, don't you?"

"Yeah", they replied.

"How many cars have you hit today?" I asked.

"Three", they replied.

"Did any of the cars have an accident?"

"No", they responded, surprised.

I then asked each boy to imagine that he was the driver of the car: "Johnny, imagine you are driving a car. You're concentrating on driving safely so you don't run into anything. Then a water balloon splats on your windshield. How do you think that would make you feel?"

"It would scare me", Johnny replied.

"Then what might you do?" I persisted.

"I guess I could have an accident", Johnny volunteered.

"You might even run the car up into someone's garden and run over a child, maybe even one of your friends."

"Yeah, I guess that could happen …" Johnny suddenly looked concerned. He had never thought of that.

Later I sat down with Matthew and explained how important it is to make wise choices in life, to think through what you're about to do and imagine how it might either help or hurt another person. It helps to put yourself in another person's place and imagine how you would feel if that happened to you. It's especially important to teach high-need children to take time to reflect on what they're going to do before they do it.

give choices

One of the tools your child needs to succeed in life is the ability to make wise choices. The strong-willed child is not likely to accept your agenda over his without a protest. Giving choices makes compliance easier: "Which do you want to do first, pick up your clothes or put away your toys?" Be sure all the choices are acceptable to you. Letting your child decide on a course of action makes him a partner in discipline, though not an equal one, as you still are in charge of what the choices are. You are simply helping your child comply with your wishes with less hassle for yourself.

Lauren, our Miss Independence, has a "charming" way of throwing something down in a fit of temper when we tell her she can't do or have something she wants. Getting her to pick up the flung item is always a challenge. After waiting until she has calmed down, we still may be met with a "go ahead and make me" stance. So we simply give her a choice. "If you cooperate with me and pick it up, I'll cooperate with you." She has come to appreciate the concept of "cooperate" very quickly.

Your child needs to learn that choices have consequences: if a child makes a choice, he lives with the consequence, whether that consequence is pleasant or unpleasant. This ties in with helping your child take responsibility for his actions. If your child chooses to leave his bicycle in the drive, and it gets damaged or stolen, then he learns the consequence of his choice. Learning consequences is especially helpful in getting a child to obey your house rules. "Please be careful and hold your juice so it doesn't spill." The child ignores your advice and the juice spills. He then asks for a refill. "I'm sorry, you chose not to be careful and there is no more juice." The child has learned that choices have consequences. For some children, especially younger ones, too many choices can be overwhelming. In that case, limit the alternatives to two: "Would you like to wear your pink dress or your red dress?"

day care for high-need children

Many a mother has had her career plans derailed by her high-need child. Sometimes no one but parents are willing or able to keep up with the constant maintenance demanded by a high-need child. You may have to face the reality that you cannot find day care for your high-need child, yet here are some tips on trying.

Consider delaying your return to work

Is returning to work sooner rather than later a need or a want? Some mothers need to work for financial reasons; others fear if they get off the career track they may never be able to get back on; for some a career outside the home fills a real need they have.

Full-time day care was too much for my child; full-time motherhood was too much for me.

Explore your options

Having a high-need baby who is supersensitive to separation compels you to explore all your options. Can you and your partner do shift work so that your baby is cared for at all times by one of you? That can be tough on a marriage: you become ships passing in the night, and nearly all of your time is spent relating to baby instead of to each other. Still, it may be a workable short-term solution, until your child matures enough to handle separation.

Try job sharing with another mother of a high-need baby

You both share one full-time job and share the care of each other's child. If there is a high-need-child support group in your community, do some networking to see if other mothers have needs similar to yours.

Infants under one year of age will need one-on-one care, from a caregiver who either comes to your home (a nanny) or cares for baby in her home (a childminder). Not surprisingly, some high-need toddlers do well in childminding situations. They seem to be entertained by other toddlers and the older preschool children, who see them as just another playmate and not a "problem child".

I'm afraid to leave her with just anyone because I honestly am afraid she will get neglected or, even worse, shaken by someone who doesn't know her as I do.

Let your infant or child be your barometer in making your choice

If you see no concerning mood swings or un-desirable behaviours cropping up, then continue with your choice. However, follow the same guidelines you will use in selecting a school, and when in doubt, pull him out (see "Matching Child and School", page 213).

Above all, choose a caregiver who understands and believes in the reality of the high-need child, agrees with your parenting style and does not sabotage it, and seems to be a nurturing person. Ask yourself, "When I am away, is this the person I want mothering my child?" (See "Day-Care Nightmare", pages 238–41.)

let your child know what you expect

Many high-need children have an innate sense of fairness, of justice, of right and wrong. Yet their persistence, their headstrong quality, and their wanting to do things their way may be perceived as defiance when it really is not. The child is not, in effect, saying, "I won't"; she is saying, "I don't want to." To get children to want to switch from their agenda to yours, let them know exactly what kind of behaviour you expect. The home is like a mini-society. It is the first place where a child is required to conform, to obey, the first place where there are rules that need to be followed. All children, especially high-need ones, are looking for norms. How are they supposed to behave? What is expected of them? Children thrive when these expectations are clearly conveyed and reinforced. For example, children need to learn what behaviour you will tolerate and what you won't. "I don't do tantrums", you say as you walk away from a howling four-year-old. "But I really like playing with you, and I'll be in the next room when you're ready." "I don't like whining, but I do like your nice voice. Come to me when you're ready to talk in your nice voice." As a toddler Matthew loved to scream. He seemed to enjoy not only the intensity of his own voice but also the reaction of listeners as they stopped in their tracks in amazement at his powerful little voice. Rather than constantly being on his case with the "stop screaming" command, we set the house rules: "We scream only outside on the grass." We then ushered the junior tenor outside. He learned the behaviour we expected: screaming must be done outside. So, whenever he felt like screaming, he could go outside. (An alternative for people living in flats or when the weather is really nasty could be "When you want to scream, find a room with no one in it.")

We constantly try to reinforce and remind our child that some behaviour, such as rude noises, talking constantly, rough hugging, or running into people, is unacceptable and annoying to other people, and that he needs to express what he is feeling appropriately or try to talk with us rather than acting in-appropriately. We don't smack, hit, or strike David at all. We feel David is already out of control with his emotions and his reactions, and doesn't need to have physical violence modelled to him.

shaping is more important than controlling

Parents often confuse being in charge with being in control, and they feel that good disciplinarians must always be in control. Clinging to the control model of parenting will drive you crazy and set you up for constant power struggles, most of which you are unlikely to win. Think of your job as shaping your child's behaviour rather than controlling it. Unlike controlling, "shaping", means that you take your child's temperament and need level into consideration in your decision making and your style of discipline. Making this mind-set change from controlling to shaping does not mean you are weakening your authority; you are simply making your authority work for you. A wise disciplinarian is like a gardener, and the child is the garden. You can't control the colour of the flowers when they bloom or how they smell, but you can prune the plants, pick the weeds, and fertilize the soil so the flowers will bloom more beautifully. In disciplining a high-need child, you will find that you need to work in the garden daily lest the work gets out of hand.

Both the weeds and the flowers grow more vigorously in high-need children. The powerful personality of the high-need child may cause the weeds to overshadow the flowers, and people may see only the weeds. Your job is to identify and pull the weeds – those quirks in your child's temperament that will not work to her advantage – and to nurture the flowers – those extraordinary personality traits that dazzle admirers. Then the child's garden blossoms. Here is a list of shapers, verbal and body language cues that catch the child's attention, encourage the flowers in her personality to blossom, and direct her behaviour so that the weeds stay under control.

Offer encouragers. Give your child "praise phrases" that acknowledge desirable behaviour. Catching them in the act of being good is one of the best ways to shape desirable behaviour. Encouragers are like behavioural immunizations that stimulate the child toward wanting to please. Children with a fragile self-image need frequent booster shots. Children thrive when they can build and maintain an inner sense of rightness, a sense of "feeling good", or what adults call "inner peace". Children search for ways of behaving that reinforce this good feeling. They want to know what is the normal way to act in a certain situation. Much of the feeling a child attaches to a behaviour comes from the people he most values – parents and other care-givers. If these people of significance – those the child most wants to please – are tuned in to the child's behaviour and encourage desirable behaviour (along with discouraging undesirable actions), they can keep the child on the path of desirable behaviour. Once the child gets used to feeling good from hearing encouraging responses, he is motivated to continue to please. He gradually weeds out behaviours that get unpleasant responses. Eventually, the child's inner rightness provides the motivation to maintain this peaceful behaviour. See some examples of encouragers on the facing page.

Child's Actions	Parent's Response
Child puts toys away.	"Great job!"
Child comes when asked, despite impulse to protest.	"I like your choice."
Child catches self as he is about to hit his brother.	"Yesss!"
Child stops whining and talks pleasantly.	"I like your nice voice."

I've learned more about motivating children by coaching Little League baseball than I did in all my psychology courses in medical school. High-need children beam when they succeed, crumble when they fail. There is no middle emotion. Jason, a high-need child with a fragile self-image, had the capabilities to become a great baseball player but he lacked confidence. He was afraid to swing the bat for fear of missing the ball. Every time he got up to bat I would yell and encourage him, "Come on, Jason, you're a swinger." To a less temperamental child I might have said, "You're a hitter", but with Jason my goal was simply to get him to swing at the ball whether or not he hit it. If I had yelled, "You're a hitter" to him and he had missed, he would have returned to the dugout and fallen apart. By encouraging Jason simply to swing, I assured his success and thus built his confidence whether or not he hit the ball.

Whenever possible, avoid the judgmental tags "good" or "bad" when encouraging or discouraging behaviour. A hypersensitive child can mistranslate these loaded words. He concludes he's valued by his performance, "I'm good when I perform well" or "I'm bad when I fail." Avoid this self-esteem breaker.

You can often encourage your child without saying a word. High-need children are very perceptive at interpreting your body language, because you have spent years learning to read each other. An approving smile, a "thumbs-up" gesture, a wink can do wonders toward encouraging a child to continue good behaviour. He notices that you notice and he likes your approval. On the other hand, be aware that he will notice your clenched fist or clenched jaw, your pursed lips, or your eyes as you roll them upward.

Praise appropriately. You don't have to fill your child's whole day with accolades. Children can smell insincerity. Your genuine praise will lose its punch in these surroundings. Avoid gushing with praise when your child doesn't really deserve it. Often simply showing you noticed

Child's Action	Parent's Reminder
Child about to climb in a forbidden place.	"You know better …"
Child jumps up from dinner table.	"You know where your plate belongs" (as you point toward the sink).
Child is about to overwhelm a smaller playmate.	"Remember how strong you are."
Child chases ball into street.	"Ah! What do you stop and look for?" (Also, ball gets "time out" to reinforce the reminder.)

and care will win more points with your child than giving elaborate, phoney praise. This conveys to your child that desirable behaviour is simply the norm; it's nothing extraordinary, it's simply what you expect.

You may have to increase the dosage of encouragers during stretches when your child's self-image is low or when she is in a particularly negative mood. Eventually as children get used to the good feeling that accompanies good behaviour, they come to expect less praise from you and are able to evaluate and encourage themselves.

Give reminders. The busy minds of high-need children race along on their own agenda, often to the exclusion of your directives. They are so absorbed in their own activity that they don't remember the things you've told them a thousand times before. Reminders are positive cues that jog children's memory, prompting a change from their mind-set to yours. These looks and phrases are shorthand for behavioural expectations that you have previously planted in your child's mind. See examples above.

High-need children perceive reminders as non-controlling; they feel that you respect their part in carrying out the desired behaviour. When you give them part of a directive, they can fill in the blanks themselves. You have just reminded them. If verbal reminders don't work with your older child, try written reminders. Hayden responded well to Post-its strategically placed to remind her of what was expected. This way she didn't have to be confronted by us.

"Rewind" and "replay" games are helpful reminders for the forgetful and impulsive child. They are particularly useful in encouraging cooperation, especially when a child grumbles. I ask Matthew to clean up the playroom. "But Dad", Matthew grumbles. I immediately look him in the eye and say, "Rewind!" Then I take a few steps back, make a grander entrance into the room and say, "Matthew, will you please clean up the playroom?" I am giving Matthew a second chance, letting him know that his first response was unacceptable, but we're going to try it again. I expect (and get) a compliant response this time.

"Replay" is especially helpful in dangerous situations. Stephen had a habit of impulsively running out into the street, forgetting to look first. We played the replay game. Twenty-five times I ran with him toward the street, hand in hand, and we stopped at the edge of the pavement, looked both ways, said "no cars", and then continued across the street. I planted in Stephen's mind a scene that he would instinctively replay every time he ran toward the pavement. When he was five, Matthew ran through a puddle on a concrete pavement and slipped and fell. To distract him from his sore bottom and soothe his wounded self-image, we played replay. We both ran toward the water puddle, stopped short of it, went around it, and continued on. We replayed the scene several times. High-need children appreciate the energy you expend to make your point that this is the behaviour you expect, not simply a mere preference. It makes a difference between their being compliant and obstinate.

Tony has a hard time controlling his feelings. He hyper-reacts to everything. He gives the same ear-splitting scream for everything that happens to him. I didn't like not knowing whether he was badly hurt or had just a little bump. This was wearing on me, and I was afraid his friends would think his outbursts were inappropriate. So I gave him a way to rate his feelings: "From one to ten, let's give your hurts numbers, one being a little bump you can barely feel and ten being a cut with lots of bleeding so you have to go to the hospital." When he "exploded" I would quickly ask, "How much does this hurt, from one to ten?" He found the idea of rating his feelings intriguing, so he would stop and realize he was usually overreacting. I like him better this way.

Provide behaviour stoppers. One of the most useful behaviour shapers for high-need children is the time-out. This behavioural-modification technique works for most children, though not all.

A time-out is likely to work for the high-need child when it is used in a way that is non-confrontational and non-controlling. It's simply a break in the action, which gives your child a chance to change behaviour, and you a chance to plan further strategy. It's an alternative to an angry confrontation in which your temper may impair your judgment, leading you to issue discipline ultimatums that result in defiance rather than compliance.

High-need children require a personalized time-out programme, sold to them with a bit of creative marketing. For our more compliant children we simply used the term "time-out". Our high-need children perceived this term as negative and they rebelled. So, we made the request more positive: "You need Lauren time", or "Let's have some quiet time", or "Let's try some thinking time."

A time-out is not only useful to shape children's behaviour, it can be a sanity-saver for parents. Many times when children's behaviour grows annoying, Martha will simply say "I need a time-out" as she retreats to another room.

Because high-need children are ultra-sensitive and want to please, if you catch them in a particularly empathic mood, you can stop their behaviour simply by saying, "That disturbs my peace", a phrase Martha has often used successfully.

Time-outs were somewhat helpful in disciplining true behavioural acts of disobedience (throwing something, or wilfully defying a given instruction, etc.), but we had to modify these in an effort to appease Haley's temperament. My friends were sending their children to their rooms for twenty minutes, but this brought on a strong reaction from Haley. She had such strong fears, and being isolated that far from us sent her into a frenzy. We accomplished the same thing by insisting she stay in the next room, which was close enough that she could hear our voices. We also did this when her negative mood got the best of us and she needed an "attitude adjustment". In this case, she could come out as soon as she put a smile back on her face.

Provide motivators. High-need kids are highly motivated; they're just motivated in their own direction. The key to compliance is helping your child want to behave, to make your wants and the child's wants the same. Parents of high-need children become masterful motivators, pulling out just the right technique at the right moment to lead their child down the path of least resistance. They can do this because they have been practising from birth the art of getting into their child's mind, seeing the world through their child's eyes, and walking in the child's shoes. As one parent-disciplinarian said, "I walk with her awhile on her path and then gradually turn her onto my path." Motivators are creative ideas that encourage children to want to do what you want them to do. Purists would call them bribes. Here's how to get your wishes to be their wishes.

Give your child a request he can't refuse. In issuing your directive, tack his want onto yours: "Josh, finish putting away your toys so we can go to the pool." Fortunately, high-need kids are bright, and they seldom pass up an offer like this. Tacking on an incentive at the end of your request avoids power struggles and gets the job done.

Make reward charts. Reward charts and ticket systems are time-honoured techniques of motivating desirable behaviour. While generally we are not strong proponents of such behaviour-changing gimmicks, for high-need children they can be particularly useful. They tap into a child's creativity and give her a sense of participation in the process of changing her own behaviour. Charts are particularly useful to turn around a negative child. Reward systems are only temporary behaviour modifiers. They get children in the habit of having, and give them a taste of, the good feelings that go along with pleasing mum and dad. Eventually, wean the child away from the system and let good be its own reward.*

High-need children are visual and sensory and are unlikely to be motivated by vague and

---

* For step-by-step ways of constructing reward charts, see *The Good Behaviour Book* (Thorsons, 2005).

abstract promises. When we added a dog to our household, ten-year-old Matthew wanted the job of feeding him. However, Martha had the ultimate responsibility to make sure it got done, and she got tired of having to supervise. So she put up a checklist for Matthew to use. All he had to do was check off the day once the feeding was done; but then he'd forget to use the checklist even when he did feed the dog. Right around this time Matt asked for a new Boogie Board for the beach. So Martha brought one home and presented it to Matt, but told him it had to stay in its packaging, unused, sitting in his room, until he was able to remember to check off dog feeding for fourteen consecutive days. He had to start over twice, but he was motivated not only by the lure of the waves but also by the sight of that brand-new board. Already having the board in his room, rather than merely promised, made Matthew even more eager to get it to the beach. Of course, the way to do that was to feed the dog faithfully and comply with Martha's check-off system. Matthew was able to get himself into the habit of remembering to do his job on his own.

Natural rewards. High-need children generally appreciate the logical consequences (natural rewards) that go along with good behaviour or following family rules. "When you learn how to play nicely with one friend, then we can invite more friends over", a mother promised her child to lessen toy squabbles during playtimes. "When you put the first toy back where it belongs, then you can play with another one", said the father to the daughter who had a habit of trashing the playroom. Most high-need children respect the natural, logical consequences that accompany desirable behaviour.

Capitalize on a high-need child's sense of justice. Try what we call the "give-and-take" system of rewards. To discourage undesirable behaviour, take away something (e.g., tickets or coins); to reinforce desirable behaviour, give something to the child.

I have found the chart system very effective in getting my six-year-old to complete his jobs without a hassle. Now, instead of grumbling, he completes each job and marks it off. If he completes each job without needing a reminder, he earns a sticker for the day and a special treat at the end of the week. Rewarding positive behaviour really works! To discourage undesirable behaviour, such as arguing, refusing to obey, whining, and "toilet talk", we take the opposite approach. First, we clearly explain what behaviour we will not tolerate. Each "infraction" costs a penny, payable immediately from his bag of twenty pence he got at the beginning of the week. We simply say, "You're arguing, that's a penny." If the behaviour continues or he protests, he forfeits another penny. He receives a new bag of pennies every week. Whatever is left over at the end of the week goes into his piggy bank. The number of pennies he gets to keep is steadily increasing, and even he admits it pays to cooperate.

chapter 13

how to talk to and listen to the high-need child

High-need children are needy communicators. These perceptive kids are very good at reading faces. Their supersensitive radar is constantly taking readings of the emotional climate around them, how it affects them, how they can share in it, and how they can fix it if not to their liking. These kids think deeply.

These communication characteristics, like so many other high-need traits, have a better or worse effect on the roller coaster of living with a high-need child. For the better, they are expressive, caring, empathetic, and are literally "touched" by an equally sensitive parent communicator. For the worse, they are deeply bothered by rage, anger, and any verbal or body language that threatens their well-being.

Laura watches me like a hawk to detect my mood. She wants to be on my wavelength, to be tuned to my emotional dial. One day she looked at me and said, "Are you happy with me?" "Yes, I am happy with you, and I'm happy with myself", I responded.

The attachment style of parenting we describe in Part I gives parents a head start on communicating with their high-need child. The mutual sensitivity to each other's emotions sets up the parent and child to be able to read each other. Attachment parenting produces good communication. Whether it's a discipline situation or simply having fun, good communication is the recipe for smooth family living. In this chapter we'll discuss ways to keep this communication going.

understand your child's viewpoint

High-need children are so caught up in what they want, what they need, and the importance of their own agenda that they become parent-deaf very easily. In communicating with power-kids remember the power of the spoken (and unspoken) word to either support or tear down ego strength. Creative communication gets the child's attention in a positive way, making compliance more likely. Nothing wins over a high-need child like feeling that you truly understand his position. Try these respectful communication tips.

Get behind the eyes of your child. High-need children have strong preconceived ideas about the way they want things to be. If Susie expects the jam to be on top of the peanut butter and you absentmindedly serve the reverse, expect either Susie or the sandwich to hit the floor. You will save yourself a mess to clean up and a two-year-old to calm down if you rewind the scene and play it again.

Very small things can make him hysterical. For example, if he wants to turn off the light and I do it instead, he will break out into huge, convulsive tears. It does not matter that I did not know he wanted to turn off the light.

Reverse and say, "Oh, I'm sorry, you wanted to turn off the light", flip the switch on, and then let him do it. This way you have modelled to him that words can be used to fix a very distressing situation. This is not "catering" to your child, it's preserving your sanity while preserving your child's need to feel powerful. The high-expectation stage will eventually pass and your child will become less rigid in his expectations. Sometimes you may have to go into "rewind" to detect what set your child off.

One day George dropped a crayon as we were walking across a car park. I had forgotten he had the crayon. He sat down and started crying. I thought he had decided he did not want to hold my hand anymore, so I picked him up and carried him. He was screaming and crying and throwing a total fit. I could not get him locked into his car seat. He was screaming that he wanted something, but I could not understand what he was saying. Finally, I took him back to where the whole problem had started, where I found the crayon. As soon as we found it, he was fine.

Give advance notice. "We will be leaving soon. Say bye-bye to the toys, bye-bye to your friends …"High-need children do not transition easily and need time and patience to switch from their agenda to yours. Respect their intensity.

Speak your child's mind. Showing empathy appeals to the child's sense of justice. High-need children are likely to be more compliant when they truly feel that you appreciate their viewpoint, even if you don't agree. Show that you understand what's going on in your child's mind. "You really want that toy, don't you? It must be very hard to say no to yourself." Let the child vent her feelings for a while until the intensity of the desire wears out a bit.

Keep your directives non-threatening. High-need children are quick to retaliate if they feel attacked. Instead of "You'd better clean up this mess", try "I would like to help you clean this up."

getting your child's attention

Remember, high-need children are often so engrossed in their own agenda that they have difficulty switching from theirs to yours. It takes more than calling from three rooms away to get their attention. Try these attention-getting techniques:

Connect before you direct. Make eye-to-eye contact with your child to get her attention. Teach her how to focus on you: "I need your eyes" or "I need your ears." For the child who is especially absorbed in her own ways, it helps to squat down to her height. Hold one or both of her hands, or put one or both of your hands on her shoulders and square her off toward you, so that your eyes meet. High-need children know what they need for their well-being and enjoy the feelings they have when their being is well. So they strive for communication skills that maintain this feeling. Listen to them. You want your body language and tone of voice to convey, "What I have to say to you is important and I need your undivided attention." Make your facial expressions caring, smiling, and happy. If a child perceives your attempts to connect as angry and controlling, she is likely to withdraw. You want her to perceive that what you have to say will be of interest to her.

Use the child's name, please. Beginning your request with the child's name shows the child that you value him as an individual, and it gets his attention. High-need children particularly like to hear their names. Pause a few seconds between the child's name and your directive, giving your child time to click out of his agenda and listen to your request: "Johnny – please help mummy set the table."

Settle the upset child. When high-need children are upset they tend to get so caught up in their own emotions that they can't hear your request. Try to restore the child's emotional equilibrium with kind, soothing words, a hug, some holding, or whatever assistance settles the child into a mood where she can listen to what you have to say.

holding your child's attention

Because high-need children are so imaginative, it's often difficult for them to focus on what you have to say. Their minds are racing forward to what they want to do. So it's not only challenging to get their attention, it's equally challenging to hold it. Try these focus-holding suggestions:

Keep it brief. In issuing a directive to a high-need child, stick to the one-sentence rule. Try to state the request in one simple sentence. Children tend to tune out elaborate explanations of what is required of them. Often one parent can get quicker responses from high-need children than the other can. Parents who try to deal with the child's feelings about a proposed action tend to ramble on, sometimes taking several minutes to issue a directive. Other parents get right to the point. Here's an example. A five-year-old and seven-year-old were using little trinkets called pogs as play money to bet on how fast their toy racecars would go. Mother intervened, explaining why she didn't want them to bet. She went on to explain what was wrong with the whole principle of gambling. The children quickly tuned out mum's lecture and kept on playing the game. Father stepped in: "Gambling is illegal. This looks like gambling to me. Give me your pogs." Most high-need children have an uncanny sense of fairness and logic, and this father's clear and logical way of communication got immediate results.

In our home, Martha is the communicator, but sometimes her skill is no match for Erin's determination to win. Matthew has this same quality, though he is not quite as practised. Erin has three more years of experience. They both know that Martha has the patience to explore many angles of a proposed action and that, in doing so, they may hit on an angle that could cause her to change her mind and say yes. (This is one reason why some parents avoid saying yes or no initially, but rather "I'll think about it and let you know when I decide.") There are times when Martha realizes at the outset that her answer needs to be no and she'll send the case directly to me because I'm very good at saying simply "I'm sorry, but the answer is no. That would not be good for you." Father has spoken. End of case. Mother is grateful.

Keep it simple. The younger the child, the fewer the syllables, and the shorter the sentence. To be sure your request sinks in, ask your child to repeat it back to you. If he can't, it's too complicated.

Don't be a buzz saw. When the child gets older you can write down your requests, so you can avoid being seen as a nag.

Watch the body language. During your discipline conversation, watch your child's eyes to see if his attention is wandering. If he has that glazed look, offer reminders: "Johnny – I still need your eyes", "Mary – I still need your ears."

Give one directive at a time. Some creative children have a mind so full of their own ideas that there is little room for anything else. They literally forget what you tell them. Instead of a long list: "Brush your teeth, wash your face, put on your pyjamas, and pick out a bedtime story", issue these requests one at a time. After the child has accomplished the first task ("Brush your teeth"), remind him of the next ("Now wash your face"), and so on.

Keep the dialogue two-sided. If you ramble on without giving your child a chance to respond, his attention is likely to wander. During the conversation, stop and ask your child questions ("Did you understand?") or invite his comments ("What do you think?"). This helps hold his attention and helps him participate in the discipline process.

encourage compliance before defiance

As you are telling your child what you want him to do, the child is already trying to decide if he wants to comply. Try to issue the directive in a way that will help the child's mind-set get on track with yours.

Substitute and distract. As you remove the dangerous object clutched in your toddler's hands, offer something safe yet still interesting. For example, trade the scissors for a wire whisk in a plastic bowl.

Prohibit and provide. When saying no to one thing, give your child an alternative that he will like: "You may not cut with the sharp knife, but you may cut with the table knife"; "You may not play across the street, but you may play next door."

Give choices. Before you open your mouth, be clear that all the alternatives are equally acceptable to you. Then offer a simple choice: "Do you want to wear your blue shirt or your red one?" "Do you want to brush your teeth first or put on your pyjamas first?" Power-kids need choices. Sharing in the selection process, besides encouraging compliance, makes them feel important.

Stay positive. Hearing "no" puts the child on the defensive and immediately prompts him to dig in his heels and hold fast to his position. Instead of "Don't write on the furniture", say, "Here, write on this" and hand your child a pad of paper or an old envelope. Instead of "No throwing the ball in the house", try "You may throw the ball outside." If you need immediate compliance because of a dangerous situation, shout the child's name: "Lauren!" This stops the child in her tracks and lets her think about the wisdom of her action. Then she is likely to redirect herself or be redirected.

Help the child save face. Appeal to the child's self-esteem. A mother brought her high-need child in for counselling. He had a fragile self-esteem and was ultra-sensitive toward any perceived put-downs. During our interview Johnny started hanging on an expensive baby scale in my surgery. My impulse was to save my scale and let Johnny's fragile self-esteem fall where it may, but the mother quickly intervened. "Johnny, please get off the scale", she said, adding, "because you're so strong." The child immediately complied. His mother's wisdom and her sensitivity toward him helped him follow her order and not lose face.

Convey your need, also. Begin your directive with "I need." Instead of "Stop running", say, "I need you to stop running around the house" or "I need you to help Mummy now." These directives work well if your child is in the mood to want to please you. Helping you gives the child a reason to comply.

Convey the behaviour you expect and quickly add a reward. Use the "when-then" form of communication. "When you finish picking up your toys, then you can play outside." "When" implies that you expect the child to obey. It works better than "if", which suggests that the child has a choice. Also, starting with the "when", the thing the child has to do first, helps him put the upcoming events in proper order. Preschoolers especially need this help with sequencing.

Let the child mess up. Persistent kids often have to learn the hard way. The good news is they are bright enough to learn from their mistakes. When your child ventures into a task you are absolutely certain won't work, your instinct is to spare her the frustration of failing. Sometimes it's best to offer your child your opinion and then let her learn from the consequences. Our three-and-a-half-year-old, Lauren, insisted on pushing her baby buggy filled with dolls down a long hill to the beach. I knew that she would soon tire of this venture, especially since she'd have to push it back up the hill, and I tried to convince her to take along a more manageable toy. It became quite clear that her mind was made up, and she would not consider any alternatives. So down the hill she trekked, baby buggy pulling her along. Halfway down the hill she realized she had made a mistake and also realized that I was not about to rescue her. When it came time to return, she realized she'd have to push the baby buggy back up the hill. It wasn't necessary for me to preach an "I told you so" sermon, as my body language gave her the message that either she had to push the baby buggy back up the hill or the buggy stayed at the beach. She arrived home an exhausted but wiser child.

Listen creatively. In communicating with a high-need child it is very important to learn how to listen. Persistent kids tend to be opinionated, even if their viewpoint defies natural laws. Our preteen, Erin, who is destined to be a trial lawyer, once pleaded her case for why she absolutely had to have a certain outfit (which really was a mismatch and much too expensive). We listened attentively as she put forth all of her reasons why the outfit was important to her. We nodded appropriately, interjecting periodic supportive comments ("I understand ... you really like that dress ...") so that she knew we understood her reasoning. We let her vent while gradually throwing in subtle objections, finally adding, "Is that really the way you want to spend your baby-sitting money?" As the dialogue wound down, Erin literally talked herself out of her own wish. We had simply nudged her a bit.

guide your child toward the conclusion you want

Remember, high-need children are often impulsive and act before they think. Try to help them think through what they're doing so that they themselves come to the same conclusion that you have about the desired course of action.

By telling your child to take some "thinking time", you give her the opportunity to re-think her unacceptable behaviour. This is sort of a time-out: "I want you to sit there and think about what you did." Avoid asking a child, "Why did you do that?" Most children don't know why they do things and you're unlikely to get an answer. Better is "Let's talk about what you did."

If your four-year-old is flinging his toys around the living room, instead of ordering, "Pick it up!" sit next to the mess and ask your child, "Where does this belong?" After he answers, add, "Let's go put it there. Then it will be easier to find your toys when you need them."

Persistent kids are preoccupied with their agenda and resist alternatives. The key to turning their choice into yours is to let them think it is their choice. Our three-year-old would balk whenever I said, "Lauren, hold Daddy's hand while we cross the street." Martha got immediate compliance by saying, "Lauren, help Mummy across the street." Or, "Hold my handbag strap."

model control

High-need children are prone to outbursts of anger, tantrums, and shouting when they don't get their way, or when they need to vent frustration. It's tempting to join them or yell louder and overpower the child. This seldom works. Try these alternatives:

"Use your words." When a child is throwing a tantrum, softly and respectfully look him in the eyes and ask him to "use your words and tell Daddy what you need". Often simply stopping to find words to express emotions will diffuse a tantrum.

I help her learn how her body feels when she is upset, what kinds of behaviour are appropriate ways of expressing her emotions, that it's okay to feel those things, and I especially let her know that I really do understand how she feels. The reason I can say that is that through parenting Melissa, I have realized that I am a high-need person too. I have a unique temperament that is not always appreciated, especially since I was never taught to express it appropriately. I had to learn that on my own as an adult. These children are so misunderstood by society and even by their own parents. I hope every parent can learn to understand their spirited youngsters so they can then pass that understanding on to everyone else who deals with them, such as teachers, day-care providers, and relatives.

The louder the child, the softer the parent. As your child is venting his emotions, expressively, in the manner of high-need children, interject suitable empathizing remarks: "What would you like me to do?" or "I understand." The soft, understanding, caring adult voice along with a comforting touch will often wind down the yelling child until he collapses into your arms.

We tried a new concept called "I need a hug" to combat Haley's anger and frustration levels. When Haley was at her angriest she would lash out verbally and become unmanageable and, quite honestly, unlikable. I'm convinced it was linked to her feeling of being out of control, but I knew that something had to be done because this anger turned the whole house upside down. I realized that many times her anger was a call for help and if we could arrest the anger before it

matching child and school

High-need children are different. High-need children can be challenging. Thus, many of these children enter school with the odds stacked against them. Many high-need children learn differently, they respond differently to authority figures, and they respond to peers differently. How a child feels about his performance at school and his being accepted by peers greatly affects his self-image, which in turn influences his desire to learn. A child who feels good about himself is more likely to do well in school. A child who feels less confident, often because of a mismatch between child and teacher or child and school, will not develop a healthy attitude about learning or about life. Here are some practical things parents can do to help their child achieve the two goals of education: developing tools for learning, and building a good self-image and a good attitude toward lifelong learning.

Do your homework
Before enrolling your child in a school, visit it, get to know its overall philosophy, and talk to parents whose high-need children have had the teacher your child will have. If you have a choice of teachers for your child, meet with all of them prior to school entry, observe their classrooms in action, and use your best parent's intuition to decide, "Is this the person I want teaching my child?"

My child has needed a high level of everything since the day she was born. She seemed to be constantly in my arms for the first year; she weaned at three years; she slept in our bed until age five. Needless to say, where she went to school and who would be her teacher were major decisions for us. I really wasn't afraid of her going to school because down deep I knew that she was a solid and secure child who could handle the challenges of school, yet I wasn't going to take any chances. I arranged for her to have a teacher whom she had met several times and knew. I also arranged for her to be in the same class as her friend. I made a point of being a frequent volunteer at the school and of going on all the field trips. I am happy to report that she was much loved by the teacher, who called her "the best-adjusted child in the class". She was also liked by her peers and was a straight-A student. Yet, school was not always a positive experience for her. During particularly difficult times or years I home-schooled her.

Be sure child and teacher fit
You may find it tough to find the teacher who strikes the right balance between nurturing and educating. Look for both.

I was so reassured by the teacher's caring attitude that I didn't pay attention to how little my child was being taught. In an effort to put

Susan into a nurturing environment, I had underestimated her desire to learn. I soon realized that she needed to be challenged for her to stay "plugged in". My fears had led me to get Susan into a safe, nurturing school. I discounted her abilities. We feared that if a school were too highly structured and had expectations that were too high, it would be difficult for Susan. Yet we found that the class we chose had no structure and no expectations.

• • •

When September arrived, the teacher of our dreams entered our lives, and this year proved to be a turning point for Haley. Mrs B understood that children process information differently. She taught with a lot of word pictures, visualizations, and soft music every morning as the kids settled into their work. She was very specific with her instructions and expectations. This was the setting that Haley needed. Feeling loved unconditionally by Mrs B, Haley had the freedom to be herself, unusual temperament and all. Haley and Mrs B were a good fit and my daughter soared academically and socially.

Help your child adjust

Remember, one characteristic of high-need children is that they don't transition well. Going from home to school is a stressful transition for many children. Expect a temporary regression and some mood swings when your child begins school. Some of this is due to the different expectations that your child is now required to meet and the lower level of tolerance teachers and peers have for unusual behaviour. If you are concerned about how your child is adjusting, set her up for some "play therapy", and you'll know soon enough.

"Acting out" her day helped Karen get used to school. After school, she played school and imitated her teacher. She converted her walk-in cupboard into a classroom. We gave her an old white board that my husband had used for seminars, and she was ecstatic. She would act out the part of her kindergarten teacher (complete with silk blouses and high heels), whom she viewed as being harsh at times, and would act toward her "students" the way she saw herself being treated. This gave us a wonderful opportunity to talk about how she felt when Miss H treated her like that. Playing school was therapeutic for her. It allowed her to work out a lot of her worries through play, and actually helped her to be more ready for the next year of school.

When in doubt, take your child out

As we have repeatedly advised, don't persist with a bad experiment. High-need children often process information differently. They usually need a lot of visual aids and do best in a structured yet flexible environment. High-need children are more likely to need one-on-one attention, and many of these children are little perfectionists who fear not doing things perfectly and failing to meet the teacher's expectations. They often feel more free to "mess up" or misbehave in front of mum, a basic fact of child rearing that explains why some children perform better for teachers than parents and why others fall apart from the pressure outside their home. High-need children are likely to be ultra-sensitive about school because they equate their performance with their value as a person. High-need children, like all children, need the right balance between academics and nurturing. Since high-need children tend to be brighter, they also tend more to become bored in school. A bored child will deviate into undesirable behaviour and be labelled as a troublemaker. A high-need child who is not getting enough nurturing may become anxious and start seriously disliking school. If, after a few weeks, the nice child you sent to school on the first day is not the person who comes home every day, take this as a sign that you need to make a change.

When kindergarten started, we hoped Kerry would find a structured environment, in which we knew she would do well as long as it was accompanied by a nurturing teacher. It wasn't long before she started showing signs of regression. She became more aggressive and negative at home. After sitting in on her class, I saw the problem. The teacher was tall, intimidating, and never had been married. She had little warmth in her disposition and attitude. She had structure but no flexibility,

and had expectations that Kerry was having a hard time meeting. She had a harsh voice, even when speaking to me. And it soon became obvious to me (and to Kerry) that Kerry was not one of the teacher's favourites. Because of the way the teacher singled her out when she disobeyed, other kids in the class were also picking up cues that Kerry was undesirable. Kerry began having constant stomach aches, night waking, constipation, and didn't want to go to school. We had a conference with the teacher, who felt that Kerry needed to conform to her rules. In her eagerness to please this teacher, Kerry became an annoyance in the classroom. She was having more time-outs and was becoming more frustrated. We considered changing schools or classes, but being first-time parents we didn't want to rock the boat. In retrospect, I wish we had pulled her, but I didn't have the confidence then that I have now.

Start gradually
Going from home to school is a major change. After you have decided the when and where of schooling, start gradually. While some children plunge right into a full day or full week of school, high-need kids usually need a more gradual introduction. While you may need your child to go to school for a full day, your child may be ready for only a half day. Since behaviour often deteriorates in the afternoon hours, most high-need children do best in morning preschool nursery or

kindergarten (unless, of course, you wish to enjoy your child during her best times of the day and let the teacher handle the worst). You may need to "go to school" a few hours a day in the early weeks as your child gets accustomed to being there.

To help him get acclimatized to his first school, I stayed and knitted.

As we have repeatedly stressed, because of the mutual sensitivity between high-need children and their parents, these kids catch your moods very easily. If you are anxious about your child going to school, your child will likely also be anxious. Moods between parents and child are contagious, especially between high-need children and high-touch parents. Give your child the message that school is fun, you're excited about it, and it's okay to be there.

High-need children will tax the creativity of their teachers just as they do their parents', so it's important to make certain the teacher and the child are a good fit and to continue to monitor the effect of the school on your child's intellectual and emotional growth.

raged, we could halt the vicious cycle that would inevitably end up with tantrums and screaming in her room. I explained to Haley that I really thought she was old enough and smart enough to "play a new game" with Mummy. It was called "I need a hug." I told her that when she started feeling angry, discouraged, or frustrated she should come and tell me that she "needed a hug". I told her that hugs were beneficial to all of us and that they helped to calm us down and make us feel good about ourselves. What a change! Many times a day, especially on the most trying ones, Haley will find me and put out her arms. It took a few months of practice, but it is a valuable tool we still use today, and the results have been marvellous.

use proper body language

Good communication between parent and child doesn't mean you have to be talking all the time. Capitalize on your child's sensitivity toward your body language. If you are deeply connected, sometimes just the look on your face or the tone of your voice will be enough to bring your child's behaviour into line. Get your child used to reading your body language and use these subtle reminders to prompt a quick change of behaviour before trouble escalates. High-need children are especially sensitive to facial gestures. Develop a firm, yet respectful "I mean business" look and a tone of voice that conveys, "I'm the parent, you're the child, this is the behaviour I expect, end of discussion." Don't feel that you have to walk on eggshells and always worry about damaging little psyches when communicating with your children. Sometimes you simply have to pull rank: Johnny, I want your toys picked up, *now.*

acknowledge your child

Include your child in the flow of conversation. In the presence of a child, seldom talk about the child in the third person, like you would a pet. This devalues the child. For example, when your spouse comes home, instead of saying, "Guess what great grades Michael got in school today?" try, "Michael, tell Daddy what great grades you got in school today." Don't steal the child's thunder. While parents should delight in what their children do, let the child share the storytelling, and the glory. After all, he has first bragging rights. Talk with your child, not about your child. This invites your child to connect.

chapter 14

the payoff – for children
and for parents

"It's been a long, tough struggle, but we're finally beginning to cash in on our investment", said Susan and John, parents of high-need child Amy. Since our interest in high-need children began in 1978, we have had the opportunity to observe these children growing up and the long-term effects on their parents.

Because high-need children are keenly perceptive and delightfully sensitive, they notice things, and these things that they see, hear, and feel become part of themselves. While you cannot take all the credit or all the blame for how your child turns out, the style of parenting you practise and the daily living you model to your child do have long-term effects. We have observed that there is a payoff when you practise the responsive style of parenting we advocate throughout this book.

High-need children show many wonderful qualities, and while not all high-need children who have received responsive parenting show these good outcome traits all the time, most of the children show most of these traits (and others we've mentioned elsewhere in this book) most of the time.

empathy

These are *kids who care*. From birth on, these children were on the receiving end of nurturing. Someone cared for them. Caring, giving, listening, and responding to needs became the family norm, and these qualities became part of the child. The child went from receiver to giver. When friends are hurting, these children rush to help. These are compassionate kids who hurt when other people hurt.

Studies on troubled teens and psychopaths have shown that these people have one abnormal feature in common: a lack of caring. They feel no remorse for what they do. They act without considering the effects of their behaviour on others. Not so the high-need children who are the product of attachment parenting. These children consider the feelings of others before they act, even though many of these children by nature are impulsive. They care about how their actions affect other people. They have a healthy sense of guilt, feeling wrong when they act wrongly and feeling good when they should. Connected kids care.

sensitivity

Because these children are on the receiving end of sensitive parenting, they become sensitive themselves. These children grow up with a deep inner sense of rightness. They are keenly aware when this rightness is upset and they strive to bring things back into balance. As teens they are deeply bothered by social injustice. Our older children are quick to notice when we are guilty of domestic injustice toward the younger ones.

I watch these children in playgroups. These early takers have become good givers. They actually share willingly – something that is difficult for many children. In playgroups, they are concerned about the needs and rights of their peers as they've seen that modelled.

These children are more sensitive to their friends and to their parents. High-need children are supersensitive to your moods. When you feel stressed, they act stressed. Eventually, this sensitivity becomes an asset, so that when you feel bad they act their best (just the opposite of what they used to do) in order to help you feel better. I have witnessed our own children and others trying to console their upset parents,

"Don't cry, Mummy, I'll help you" or "It's okay, Daddy, I love you." Watching a sensitive three-year-old console the adult she loves is one of the most beautiful payoffs you will ever witness. No adult therapist could ever offer words that have such impact as those that naturally flow from the heart of a sensitive child.

As an added bonus, because you were sensitive to your child, you will find your overall sensitivity to everyone and everything else goes up a notch. The ability to get behind the eyes of your child, to see things from his viewpoint, to think, "kid first" carries over to your sensitivity to your mate, your friends, your job, and your overall social awareness.

sense of justice

Because of their empathy and sensitivity, these children have a strong sense of justice. Because they are easily bothered when this inner sense is disturbed, they are likely to fight for their own rights and for those of others. These are not wimpy kids. They will swim upstream to fight a harmful social current. The world needs these kids. Imagine if many of these high-need children grew up to be politicians and voted with their convictions rather than doing what was politically expedient.

awareness

These kids are keenly aware of the people and events around them. Their antennae are always up. The toddler whose intense curiosity was nurtured and channelled becomes the aware child and adult. He is tuned in to the world around him, and gleans from his environment those things that are to his advantage. These kids are not distant. I watch them play and socialize. They connect with people. One of the most frequent comments parents volunteer is, "She's a real people person!"

intimacy

Attachment-parented high-need children have the ability to feel close to another person, because these "Velcro babies" spent the most formative months of their lives in arms and at breast. These kids have learned to bond to people rather than to things. They become high-touch people even in a high-tech world.

Therapists whose offices are filled with former high-need children who didn't get responsive parenting tell us that most of their energy is spent in helping these people get close to someone. These people have difficulty getting connected. They do not have the capacity for feeling close. Not so high-need children who are the product of high-giving parents. These children thrive on interpersonal relationships. Being connected is their norm. The high-need infant is more likely to become the child who forms deep friendships with peers and the adult who enjoys deep intimacy with a mate. These are deep children, capable of deep relationships. Because they were close to their parents and caregivers, they become capable of strong attachments. Intimacy becomes their standard for future relationships. These children are affectionate. The connected child has learned to give and receive love.

confidence

"Confidence" comes from two words meaning "with trust". High-need children whose parents respond freely to their needs grow up as if "trust" is their middle name. They grow up learning that it is safe to trust others, that the world is a warm and responsive place to be, that their needs will be appropriately identified and consistently met. The trust they have in caregivers translates into trust in themselves.

I felt he would never leave my arms, but when he became two, he often said, "My do it." I know this is a phrase that many mothers dread (because it takes five times as long for the child to accomplish a simple task), but to the mother of a clingy baby, this phrase is a joy. Now that Jonathan is absorbed in trying things himself, he is rapidly leaving many of his old baby needs, such as demanding to be carried everywhere and never leaving my lap. I must admit that there are times when I miss being the exclusive interest in his life. But when one of those moments arises, all I have to do is give him a big hug and he stops doing what he is doing and returns to me. Mostly, I am proud to see him growing into a happy, loving, self-confident little person, especially when I realize he has done it on his own. I have simply given him the support he needed.

expressiveness

Let's face it, no matter how intelligent a person is, much of success in life depends on the ability to express oneself. A person can have great thoughts, but the ability to express them is what counts. Because their zest for life was appreciated early and their loud cries met with sensitive responses, high-need children grow up learning how to express themselves comfortably. Parents who achieve the right balance, neither ignoring the child's signals nor rewarding him for exploding, help their children learn to express their emotions freely, but appropriately. These children learn that it is okay to have and express feelings, but that they must consider the feelings of others as well.

High-need kids tend to grow up to be talkers. This is the type of person who keeps a party lively. Society is much more interesting because of these highly expressive kids.

persistence

Persistence and expressiveness are a dynamic personality duo. Children with these qualities know how to get their point across. These children have firm convictions and the strong personality to persist until they get their way. They believe in themselves and insist on others believing in them also.

The infant who cried incessantly until you picked him up, the toddler who kept nagging until his needs were met, and the child who exhausted your reserve by constantly asking why

reacting to danger

The key to living with high-need children is learning how to use their traits to your (and the child's) advantage. High-need children are perceptive. They are sensitive to your emotions. In a dangerous situation, the child looks to you to mirror to him, "How am I suppose to react?"

Our high-need child Lauren, even at the young age of three, is a master reader of facial expressions. One evening Lauren grabbed a piece of fish before we were able to remove the bones and got a large bone lodged in the back of her throat. She immediately communicated a "hurt throat" and had the facial expression that was telling us what the problem was. Being a paediatrician and nurse, we knew how dangerous this situation could potentially be, and we also knew the importance of keeping the muscles of the throat relaxed. Martha looked at Lauren and communicated a "You will be okay, we will help you" message in a calm and reassuring voice. Lauren picked up on how she was supposed to react and relaxed, opening her mouth, allowing me to scoop out the fish bone.

can, if this strong personality trait has been channelled appropriately, use it in leadership positions as an adult. "Persistence" is the word that comes to mind when we want to describe in a positive way our child who is the most stubborn. Erin believes strongly in herself and in her goals. If we are having a hard time seeing a vision she has for herself, she can be relentless in presenting her view.

I could hold her only the way she wanted. Everything had to be her way or no way. Today my high-need child has more character than five children combined. She is so intelligent and witty.

interdependence

The baby you couldn't put down, the toddler who clung to you, and the child who shadowed you wherever you went gave you no hint that independence would ever be her strong point. Yet, in our experience, these children grow up to have a healthy independence. Notice we stress

resource-full

High-need children who grow up in a responsive family eventually learn to use their character traits to their advantage. In the early years, when these children seem so unmanageable, parents put a lot into them: holding, comforting, redirecting impulses, and so on. Now these children have the tools to manage themselves.

healthy independence, because the Western view of independence is often not all that healthy. A high-need child who is forced to become independent never learns to use the resources of others to his advantage for a better outcome. A more useful goal is interdependence, which combines both the drive to accomplish a feat and the wisdom to ask for help to do it better. Steven Covey, author of the best-selling *Seven Habits of Highly Effective People*, stresses that interdependence is characteristic of the most successful people. High-need children who are the product of responsive parenting have learned from infancy on to use adult resources to get what they need. And because they grew up in a responsive environment, they were comfortable doing so. This becomes their standard. The ability to know when to seek help and how to get it is a valuable skill for life. High-need children who grow up in a responsive environment become interdependent adults.

ability to make wise choices

Success in life depends on making wise choices. It's easy for the emotions of high-need children to overwhelm them, causing their reasoning to shut down and get in the way of their making good decisions. Because you have taught your child to manage his emotions and to channel them to work to his advantage, he is better able to think through what he is about to do, to consider the effects of his behaviour on others and the consequences of his choices. This child is well on his way to becoming a responsible adult.

future parenting skills

Children grow up searching for a norm for everything in life, especially what it means to be a parent. By holding your infant a lot, calming her cries, responding to her needs, and practising the overall style of attachment parenting, you have modelled parenting skills for your child and shown him that this is the way parents take care of children. You are bringing up someone else's future mother, father, wife, or husband. The standard of care your child receives is one he or she is likely to carry on with the next generation. Parenting a high-need child is truly a long-term investment.

She is so sweet and maternal around babies. She is interested in babies and is always gentle with them. Her favourite toy is her baby doll, whom she lovingly carries and rocks; and even changing nappies. When I see her baby-dancing with that doll just like I did with her, I can see that all the effort with Alex during her first year has paid off. Alex won't have to read a lot of books on baby care when she is a mother. She will already know how to take care of a baby.

Not only will your child cash in on your investment in responsive parenting, you will too. Consider what we call the "need-level concept". High-need children require a high level of giving from parents. Yet the more you give, the more you get, enabling you to give more until your giving level meets the need level of your child. Early on, this may seem like one-sided giving-giving-giving; yet as your relationship grows, you begin getting back as much as you give, sometimes more. Living with a high-need child is a life-enriching experience.

closeness

Your "Velcro baby" is unlikely to grow up to be a distant child. Parents of teens often say they don't feel close to their children. We seldom hear that complaint from parents of high-need children. The interdependent relationship we discussed above is likely to be lifelong.

Over the years, in watching the parents and high-need children who thrive together, I have noticed that these parents have learned to include their children in their discussions, addressing them by name, taking their feelings into consideration, and involving them in choices that are crucial to the children, such as school placement. This closeness did not keep the children from becoming individuals or create a clone of the parent. These parents have formed a close partnership with their children, with the right balance of authority and closeness.

ease in disciplining

In the early years, disciplining a high-need child may seem to involve a constant conflict of wits and wills. Strong-willed children don't bend easily. One of the most satisfying comments we frequently hear is "I can read her so well." A high-need child will never be putty in your hands, yet with good management she will soften with age. Because you gave your child a solid and secure foundation early on, in the later years, when the conflict of wills continues, you can take a firmer stand, and your child will go along with your judgment.

There really are some wonderful rewards for putting all that time and energy into a difficult baby. A good example in our case is the subject of discipline. One would probably expect Emily to be difficult to discipline, but I have not found that to be true. Perhaps because we have had such a close and intimate relationship, she really listens to me. I know her inside and out, and I can usually tell what she is thinking. This makes certain discipline techniques such as verbal instruction, explanation of logical consequences, and modelling (the best of all) very effective tools in teaching her about the world and her place in it.

trust

The real payoff for children and parents can be summed up in one word: trust. A growing child whose needs are sensitively responded to learns to trust his care-giving environment. The parents who respond from their heart learn to trust that they know what's best for their child. This raises the self-esteem of everyone. The child feels valued because he trusts his cues will be listened to and his needs met. The parents feel valued because, though their confidence was a bit shaky early on, it grows as they see their child mature. A mutual trust develops between parent and child.

A good indicator that we must be doing something right was her comment the other night when we were going to bed. I said, "Your mummy and daddy love you very much, you know." Her reply was "Yes, and I love myself, too." This and all her many hugs and kisses are all the reward I need.

III

stories from
the experts

Where do you go to learn about living with high-need children? Naturally, you go to the homes where these children live. You meet the parents who have walked in similar shoes to yours. You see children who have similar traits as your child's. In this part we take you into these homes to see how these parents and the high-need children they live with get along. These parents are the real experts. Motivated by the desire to do what's best for their child, these parents, largely through trial and error, have come up with a wide variety of useful parenting tips. Choose from these offerings whatever fits your family situation. Remember, regardless of a child's temperament or need level, the child still must learn to fit into the family, to adjust to "house rules". After all, the child is part of family life too.

chapter 15

survivors' stories

Here the experts speak for themselves. The most useful advice about raising high-need children comes from those who have lived with them. In this chapter, parents share their stories; their successes, their failures, their children. You can learn from their experiences. Glean from these testimonies whatever will help you on your journey with your child. These parents have been there.

too tired to get dressed

The anchor on the evening news announced the arrival of my son, Patrick Douglas. Routine births aren't normally mentioned on television, but this was during a pause for "happy talk" on the set.

I was the station's 11:00pm live reporter. I'd go anywhere, do anything to get a late-breaking news story. Why, if I'd had a microphone and earpiece that night, I would have done my own push-by-push account from the delivery suite.

It must have been a slow news night! But come to think of it, I was BIG news – nearly two hundred pounds by the time Patrick arrived. (My face was the only "unpregnant" part of my body. The cameramen had long since given up their wide-angle lenses and shot my reporting from the neck up. I covered Olympic torch relays, toxic dump sites, and gang shootings – all by night.)

When Patrick arrived, we thought he'd heard too much about the world and was yelling to go back. What a set of lungs! The boy had broadcasting in his genes. But someone failed to tell him the birth had already been announced on national television.

What kind of stress had I transmitted to my little "news buddy" – the quiet guy who rode in my lap and hung in there (literally, upside down) before the camera all those late nights for nine months?

Patrick, now appearing "LIVE!" was about to teach me the real meaning of stress – and exhaustion. He just didn't like to sleep. Yes, we'd catch the late news and the *Tonight* show together. During the day it seemed he would sleep fifteen, maybe twenty, minutes max and then begin his famous fuss-and-cry routine. I don't really remember knowing night from day.

I do remember shielding my "working" husband from taking any shifts. Patrick, I believed, was *my* job. How hard could it be? I got to stay home. Besides, I was breast-feeding Patrick, so I got to do all the feeding anyway.

If you're picturing a young woman tenderly rocking and holding her newborn to her breast, your mind's tuned to the wrong channel. Imagine clicking to a late-night, B-rated horror movie, close-up on me, alone in the dim light: my teeth are clenched. I watch the clock in fear, the minutes ticking away, knowing any second the child will awaken. And then the torture would begin – sharp, shooting pain running through my breast as his voracious gums latch onto my body. I pound my leg on the floor until the initial pain subsides, but the sores … the bleeding …

The feeding drama did have a happy ending. I finally got some professional help! But what was happening to this once competent, self-sufficient twenty-seven-year-old newswoman? I had a master's degree but I hadn't taken one lousy child-development class. Patrick would have to give me a giant crash course, everything I needed to know about babies and about life.

I thought I had it all figured out – the high-profile, high-paying career, the admiration of family and friends. Toss in a husband, a kid or two and all the trimmings, all under my control.

But then God decided to get my attention with an eight-pound ball of "high-need" baby boy.

When I quickly realized Patrick wasn't going to conform to my schedule, I learned survival skills. I depleted shop shelves of dummies. I bought and borrowed devices to strap him to my body – front, back, side – wherever – to help keep him quiet. I wore him everywhere. I wore him while making beds. I wore him cooking, cleaning, doing dishes. I wore him in the bathroom.

When I went out, this blond appendage became part of my ensemble. While other women coordinated outfits with matching shoes and handbags, I "accessorized" with Patrick. Not that I ever looked good! If Patrick wasn't burping and drooling all over me, I was leaking all over myself.

Needless to say, I didn't go out much. We lived on a lonely stretch of beach, and I was away from family and friends. When we did try to go somewhere, such as out to eat, Patrick demanded the full attention of the restaurant. He and I would end up waiting in the car, and I'd get a four-course doggie bag.

When Patrick was nearly three months old, my boss, the news director, called me. When was I returning to work? I told her I'd get back to her when I'd had a night's sleep.

Ten years have now passed, and yes, Patrick and I are sleeping through the night. Those early personality quirks now seem to be working to his advantage. He stands out as a student, musician, and athlete because he's wired with intensity and determination. At piano festivals he plays Beethoven and commands "superior" ratings. As an all-star, left-handed baseball pitcher and an all-star soccer player, he demonstrates amazing athletic talent. He even gets his picture in the local paper. Coaches call him long before the seasons start. They're already "recruiting" my baby in the fourth grade.

Patrick is highly competitive. I guess that's part of the package, too. He plays hard, feels deeply. And the tears still flow easily. Perhaps one day these qualities will produce a sensitive husband and caring father.

I never did make it back to television news. Instead, I changed priorities. And three and a half years later, after I swore I'd never have another baby, Paul Anthony came along. He was beautifully wide-eyed and peaceful. When he cried out between babblings, it was sweetly tolerable.

Sixteen months later, we were surprised by the arrival of Katherine Elizabeth. A girl! How much easier can it get? Yet when she was wheeled into my hospital room, the nurse bristled and I knew I was in trouble. "Is something wrong?" I asked politely. "Just keep her here in your room", she said. "She's disturbing all the other babies!"

Looking back on early parenthood, and seven consecutive years of dirty nappies, I'm able to smile, seeing it all in its proper light.

If sweet-natured brother Paul had come before Patrick, there's little doubt in my mind I'd still be on television today. In fact, with that extra decade of TV experience, who knows? CBS might have hired me to read the evening news for millions of viewers. Instead, I read picture books to three little people. In spite of the demanding schedule and zero-figure salary, the benefits are excellent and eternal. I've signed a lifelong contract with Patrick, Paul, Katherine, and their daddy. "It's the toughest job you'll ever love", says the military slogan, but I suspect whoever wrote that never served on the front lines and in the trenches of full-time motherhood.

I'd love to say I gave up my hard-sought news career early on because I had a burning desire to stay home with my child, but the truth is I was just too tired to get dressed.

i knew something was wrong with him

When I first had Michael I didn't know how different he was. I had never had a child before and didn't have any close friends with babies nearby. I couldn't understand why I was having so much trouble just surviving every day. It wasn't until he was six months old and I read about "high-need" babies in *The Baby Book* that everything started to make more sense.

Michael and I bonded instantly. The second he was born I held him to my chest and said, "I love you, Michael" without even thinking about it. I put him to my breast and he stayed there for almost two hours. We roomed together the first night in the hospital and then left to begin our lives together.

The first few months are still a blur. I held Michael all the time. He was content as long as I was holding him and walking but would never let me put him down. I tried pushing him in a pushchair, placing him in an automatic swing or infant seat, or riding with him in the car, but he screamed almost every time I tried. So I just kept walking and walking and walking. Sometimes I was so tired I thought I might fall asleep standing up and drop him. Everyone kept telling me to put him down or carry him in an infant seat, but I knew he wouldn't like that, so I just nodded and kept walking. Even now that he's ten months old, I still hold him whenever he needs it, which is still much of the time.

Michael has never been content lying down, except after he goes to sleep (and even then he wakes up fairly often). I had problems using the pushchair in the reclining position and rarely if ever could lay him on his back on the floor. When he was little, the only way he would go to sleep was held upright on my shoulder while I walked. Even now I need to carry him upright for five to ten minutes whenever he wakes up.

Another thing that's different about him is his need for constant stimulation. Even as a young baby he always needed to be moving, looking in a mirror, staring at lights, or playing with a rattle. He started crawling at three and a half months and started walking at eight months. We move from room to room in the house together, go outside, go shopping, and keep constantly moving. Often, after fifteen minutes in one place he gets very agitated. When I hold his hand he runs, not walks, pulling me behind him.

His nighttime cries sound like cries of pain. Also, he sits up immediately upon waking up and has almost always resisted feeding lying down. Sometimes he sounds in such pain that I need to walk him around for a while before he can go back to sleep. [Author's comment: these symptoms were clues that there was a medical cause for Michael's cries. See page 160.]

Despite all this activity, he seems to need less sleep than many babies do. He goes to bed at 10:00, wakes up several times during the night, and is often up for the day by 6:30. He does take two naps a day, but they are often short or interrupted. He is so sensitive to noise that just the sound of a car door closing across the street can wake him up. He is also sensitive to noise when he's awake. If someone sneezes or blows their nose, he can become terrified and start screaming.

His sensitivity carries over into some wonderful traits though, too. He loves interacting with people and is very social. Everyone always comments on what a joker he is and how happy he seems. He laughs easily and heartily. He is full of life and is interested in everything. He amazes me with the things he notices and the pleasure he takes in them. When he walks up to me with a huge grin on his face and his arms outstretched it melts my heart. I feel relatively content now in my role as his mother. We are really "attached" and I feel like he's helped bring out the best in my mothering techniques. I understand him well enough that I can usually meet his needs before he starts crying. What's most difficult about our situation, though, is that we have had to get to this point without much support from others. Part of this is because we moved home when Michael was only four days old, leaving friends and family behind. Part of it is also because most people don't understand what a "high-need" baby really is.

One family member has told me multiple times that I should just "put in my earplugs and let him cry." Another close relative has said, "You mean he still sleeps with you? When is he going to learn to sleep by himself?" Our previous paediatrician actually told me not to hold Michael when he was sick at six weeks because then he would expect to be held when he got well. One of the comments that hurt most came from one of my best friends who told my husband I was making up the fact that Michael was a high-need baby, even though she had seen him only once since he was born. She said that all babies can be trained and that he was "high-need" because I wasn't being a good mother.

The irony is that while these people suggest that I lessen my load by letting Michael cry or by holding him less, most of them have not been willing to help hold or take care of him so that both of our needs can be met.

At first I was resentful about my situation. I hated the lack of time to myself, thought it was unfair that my baby was so "difficult" while others around me had been given such "easy" babies. I resented my husband for his lack of understanding and support and felt inadequate because of all the things I couldn't get done. After a while, though, I realized these negative feelings were just dragging me down. I couldn't necessarily change other people's opinions, but I could take some steps on my own to make things better. I sat down one night and brainstormed about what I could do.

First, I decided to use some gift money to hire someone to clean the house every other week. Now I don't worry so much about the house and how it looks all the time. Next, I decided to find a regular babysitter for Michael so I could work on hobbies, relax, exercise, or at least have some time to myself to think for a few hours a week. It required a fair amount of investment upfront because I had to spend a lot of time with the babysitter and Michael so he would be comfortable with her when I left. Unfortunately, she quit after three weeks. She said she had never taken care of a baby with so much energy and she was too exhausted after a couple of hours with him to function the rest of the night! I feel very lucky that I have already found a replacement (with more energy!). My husband and I are also working at strengthening our family unit. We are going to counselling and we are talking about having him take on more responsibility for Michael.

These changes have helped me enjoy my time with Michael even more. I try to focus on appreciating the moment and seeing the positives in it. Just today I was shopping with Michael and he started to get frustrated because it was taking so long. He wouldn't sit in the shopping trolley and was insisting on running all over the shop. I finally decided that I had no particular reason to rush and I might as well enjoy doing a little exploring with him. He found some interesting treasures on the floor and we met a friendly person who talked with us about her grandchildren. When we got back to the shopping a little later, both Michael and I were in a much better mood.

I've also learned that I will get the most support from people who understand about high-need children. When I am feeling particularly challenged by Michael I call up a friend of mine who has also had a high-need child. She can relate and encourage me in a way that a mother of an "easy" baby never could. She is also more likely to support my parenting style. For this same reason, I have changed paediatricians.

Sometimes when I just "have" to get something done, I indulge myself and pop in a video for Michael. Before I had a child it was my goal never to use a video player as a babysitter. I still try to limit its use to less than an hour a day, but I have found it a realistic solution to a difficult situation. One video in particular seems to work well with Michael. It is called *Baby Songs*. I think he likes it because it is not too loud or confusing and it talks about life from the baby's perspective with songs like "The Day I Took My Nappies Off".

We've also come up with a whole set of activities which put us both in a good mood. Michael loves the water and it seems to calm him down, so we spend a lot of time playing at the beach, the lake, and the swimming pool. He also seems to relax best when his clothes (and nappy!) are off. So I try to give him lots of time in the nude every day, in our back garden, the bathroom, the kitchen sink, or some other safe place. Feeding is also very effective with him, and I make it a point to do so frequently. It's amazing to see him go from bouncing off the walls to nursing serenely with his eyes half open and his body curled against mine. Another thing I've realized is that I can help him calm down by relaxing more myself. I do the slow-breathing exercises I learned in childbirth classes to calm down and sometimes it reflects on him.

The relationship between Michael and me and within our family is evolving every day. What works best tomorrow may very well be different from what worked today. In any case I truly feel like I've been blessed with a wonderful, remarkable, unique baby. Sometimes I like to think about the fact that by nurturing this sensitive baby now I will one day have helped to make him a wonderful, caring, giving husband, father, and grandfather.

Three weeks ago I decided to see a paediatrician who I heard understands high-need children. In addition to believing that Michael is high-need by temperament, he diagnosed gastro-oesophageal reflux as the probable cause of Michael's painful outbursts and night waking. The first night on medication he slept six hours straight. He is still a "high-need" child in most ways, but he seems to be happier, and I know he feels more comfortable.

My key feeling about this is relief. He has gone from waking up every one to two hours a night to sleeping as long as six hours at a stretch. Although he still gets up at least twice a night, he isn't in as much pain, and I am more rested overall. His naps are a little longer and rarely interrupted. He babbles more during the day and, even though this doesn't seem possible, he has even more energy!

Right now I am also trying to deal with my frustration over the fact he wasn't diagnosed sooner. I remember that when Michael was only three months old, I told his paediatrician I thought he had abdominal pains when he woke up. The paediatrician laughed at me, said I was imagining it, and told me that all mothers say that. Over the next several months, I asked other paediatricians if they could help me find out what pain was waking Michael up at night. They all said the same thing – just let him cry. I asked Michael's doctor if there could be anything medically wrong that could cause a baby to wake up so often. He said, "No, not in the case of a baby who looks so healthy."

The lessons I have learned from this are not to undervalue my intuition about my child and to search as long as I have to find support for my parenting style. I believe a baby's cries are a sign of an unmet need. I am thankful I have finally found someone who will help me figure out why Michael is crying and address the problem instead of ignoring it.

balancing a medical career and mothering

Maisie is a high-need baby. She had full-blown colic for the first three months of her life, first evidenced two weeks after her birth with the first of many nights of four to six hours of inconsolable crying and screaming.

Her crying was often heart-wrenching. The only things that would sometimes help were carrying her in a sling and rocking her. I found that my constant carrying her offered both of us some relief; although the crying didn't seem to get much better, I sensed she knew that I was there for her.

Attachment parenting as I understand it is parenting from the heart. It is the most natural and right-feeling way to approach birth and child rearing, but it is not the easiest route. Natural childbirth takes intense preparedness, breast-feeding is demanding, sharing sleep with a baby and answering a baby's needful cries are exhausting. But the long-term rewards are without bounds.

Although the colic is now, thankfully, gone, Maisie for a long time would often wake up at various times during the night crying with a vigour reminiscent of colic. We traced this

problem to some food intolerances, particularly cow's-milk products (whey and casein), broccoli and related vegetables, strawberries, and corn. Although the elimination of these products from our diet did not lead to a "miracle" cure, we feel we have seen a slow improvement in her sleep pattern. The symptoms of the food intolerances included nervous irritability leading to severe crying, nappy rash, and cold-like symptoms.

Our daughter continues to breast-feed (mainly comfort-feeding) at the age of twenty-six months. She was breast-fed exclusively until nine months of age, primarily because she seemed to have so many food intolerances.

People ask me how I have managed the birth and raising of Maisie while studying to be a doctor. Obviously, it hasn't been easy. I wound up delaying my return to work until Maisie was fifteen months old, primarily because I had difficulty leaving her in someone else's care. I felt a tremendous need to be with her, which superseded my need to go back and finish my last year of studying. But as time passed, I was able to weigh the need to be with Maisie full-time against my desire to complete the arduous task of finishing my medical training. I wanted to give my daughter a balanced perspective in both career and mothering.

We decided that the best alternative short of my staying home full-time with Maisie was to hire a nanny who would come to our house and care for her one on one. By doing this we felt Maisie would have the consistency of a primary caregiver while we were away and also the constancy of her home environment. Our nanny was selected on her ability to provide our daughter with the same attachment-parenting environment that we had set up during the first fifteen months of Maisie's life. We had our nanny come over to our house for short stays at least one month in advance to allow her to get accustomed to our daily patterns and to allow an easy transition period for Maisie and me. Maisie has done wonderfully with these upheavals, showing no noticeable signs of any problems. I attribute this to the choice of our nannies whose style and philosophy have been so close to our own.

My work schedule necessitated Maisie's being weaned during the day, and our breast-feeding pattern switched to nighttime nursing only. I maintained this schedule until Maisie was almost two years old. However, I found that I was not effectively parenting her during the little time I had with her during the day on my days off, primarily due to my being exhausted from feeding her two to three times a night. So now we compromise; she seems to understand that the breasts are asleep during the night and day, but wake up for her to feed only to help her fall off to sleep. Even when I am on call, my husband tries to bring her into the hospital so that we can continue to have this special time together as she goes to sleep.

I think that sleeping with her has actually helped alleviate some of my seemingly never ending sleep deprivation. For instance, when she was younger, whenever she awoke during the evening, it was so simple to roll over and comfort her back to sleep. For those who worry that they are teaching their child to depend on them to get back to sleep, I say RUBBISH! Maisie is now able to easily go back to sleep by singing to herself, just as I used to do for her a few short months ago.

Because of the new demands of motherhood, career, and a new and different relationship with my husband caused by a new person in the family, I went into therapy. Of all the positive things that I could have done for myself and my family, this was probably the best. One of the things I had to let go of was trying to be the perfect mother and doctor; but perhaps it is in this very struggle that I give our child and my patients the best of all possible care. The other important point that I learned was to separate out my needs from the needs of Maisie. This has allowed me to see her as a separate, beautiful, and blossoming person apart from me, who is still a part of me.

My husband and I also go to therapy together. It allows us time to reconnect as a couple. We had become so involved in caring for Maisie that we lost sight of our own relationship. That is not the kind of example we wanted to set for our daughter. So even though she may want us to be with her every minute of every day, we have started to take time once a week to nurture ourselves, which hopefully translates into an even richer relationship with Maisie.

robbed of a month of my motherhood

When we were expecting our baby, I thought a lot about parenting styles. We had heard a lot about attachment parenting, but the idea of holding a baby constantly, feeding a lot, and even sleeping with a baby seemed much too liberal. We came across another method of parenting through classes in our church. It seemed perfect for me. It addressed our fear of losing so much of ourselves as a couple. We had seen this happen to so many parents. This method claimed we would be in control if we used a feeding schedule, didn't pick baby up for every cry, and let baby cry off to sleep. I liked that. So from the day our daughter came home, we used this method of parenting. Within three weeks, Emily had become an increasingly dissatisfied baby. One of the suggestions this particular style of parenting makes is to be sure you put the baby down to sleep awake. So we did that, but she cried because she didn't understand she was supposed to go to sleep. All she knew was that she was all of a sudden left alone. The rule is you let baby cry a little bit, so we did. She cried herself to sleep. As days progressed into weeks, her cries became very intense, turning into really big screams. I sensed that this left her in an unsettled state of abandonment.

As for me, I had come home a confident mother. I had been around babies. I wasn't totally out to lunch when it came to taking care of them. So by the end of three weeks, when she was screaming all the time, I took it personally. By the time I finally got some counselling, my confidence level had dropped down to negative, and I needed a lot of repair work.

This method of parenting really shattered my confidence. I followed it as well as I could, and it wasn't working. I didn't like the fact that she was crying herself to sleep, but the other mothers who followed this method of parenting told me, "Don't give up. Follow it." They said, yes, their babies cried themselves to sleep, but eventually they stop. You would think I might have clued in, but I was a little slow on this.

After a month of trying this parent-in-control method, I realized I had been robbed! It was not only wrong for my baby, it was wrong for me. It didn't allow me the ability to read my daughter or understand her needs. I was so busy watching the clock and trying to keep her on a schedule, as this method emphasized, that I didn't know what her cries meant. Was it a feeding cry? A pain cry? Or just a "needing her mummy" cry? Once I stopped this method of parenting, it still took me a long time to learn how to read her.

Another thing it did was instil a lot of guilt and fear in me. The class had emphasized that too much attachment parenting would create a clingy baby, so every time I spent a lot of time holding and cuddling her, I worried I was giving her too much affection and spoiling her, and that I was creating a clingy baby. But she had changed from the happy, sparkly, content baby I brought home from the hospital. I really feel that's because she felt abandoned by me in the early weeks.

During my pregnancy, I had sung to her and talked to her. I had told her everything I was saying in a journal to her. So she really had a sense of my presence, and then it stopped once she was born. I am sad, even angry, because I lost some precious time with my daughter, and she with her mummy. I've shed more than a few tears about it. I wish I had done a lot more holding, loving, and cuddling rather than watching a clock and worrying about her routine and schedule. Even my husband recently said to me, "I didn't feel right about those classes, but some of our friends were so sold on it, I let myself join the crowd. We should have listened to our hearts." Instead of a contented and independent baby (as this controlling method of parenting promised), we have a very fussy baby.

Now we wear her in a sling, I feed her whenever I feel she needs it, and, would you believe, we even sleep with her. I am feeling much more confident. I enjoy her. I spend my time loving her as much as I can. I'm beginning to see a baby laughing and cooing and enjoying her mummy. I no longer worry about spoiling her. Best of all, she gives me great joy.

a late bloomer

I guess Jordan was what you'd call a "late bloomer". From the day we brought him home, he was an absolute angel. He hardly ever cried, and when he did, his needs were quickly and easily satisfied. I had a great milk supply, he latched easily, nursed vigorously every four to six hours and slept eight to twelve hours at night, waking only briefly to satisfy his tummy. (We joke now that he was resting up for the months to come!) We thought, who were we that we had been given this miracle that was perfect in every way? Who said motherhood was so hard? I thought myself crazy for quitting my job to stay home full-time. After all, what was I going to do all day? All my chores were done by 10am when he woke; by three months all the thank-you notes for the baby gifts were written, and the anxious visitors had slowed to a trickle. I had

"nothing to do", and my precious angel only slept and ate. Around the time Jordan turned twelve weeks, I got a big case of the "I'm not needed" syndrome and diverted my attention to doing some at-home typing, sewing, crafts, and of course stacks of reading that I had all that free time for. Life was good!

Well, around the same time, it seems Jordan developed the "I need you constantly" syndrome. Of course at first I was delighted. Finally I would have the chance to try out my mothering skills. It was like someone flicked on a switch in my son. All at once, it seemed, he began sitting unaided, rolling over everywhere, inch-worming here and there, babbling, crying, and just being very active. He was no longer happy being alone or sitting still. He wanted to be rocked, carried, or nursed on a continual basis. He would sleep only in arms and then only in twenty-minute stretches. He screamed for one to two hours at bedtime and would waken only minutes after being laid down. He developed a horrendous case of thrush and would have a nursing strike at least twice a month. He cried in the bath, in the pushchair, in the car seat, in bed, in his bouncy chair, and in anyone's arms but mine. We began the merry-go-round of sleepless nights and wore a path in our hallway carpet, as he would sleep only in motion. My husband and I took shifts pacing with him, and inevitably our life became a wreck.

My husband's work, my health, and our relationship as a family began to suffer. We got to the point where we started to dislike our child and wonder if we really had been blessed with a miracle after all. I felt a great deal of anger that I had not got the good-natured child I felt I needed. After all, I had a disability, and who better deserved a laid-back child than I? Friends and relatives asked what had happened and told us we had "spoiled" Jordan by never letting him cry, feeding on demand, responding to his night waking, and responding to his every need. He probably just needed a "good cry" (like there is such a thing). He'd get over it, they said. We began the roller coaster of advice: he's hungry, he's tired, he must be in pain, he's bored, he's hot, he needs space, he must be sick, he's just a "mummy's boy", your milk must be no good, give him a dummy, give him a bottle, and so on. There was no pleasing him day or night, and rivers of tears were shed. Had it not been for the support I got from La Leche League, I am certain we would be insane. Somehow we dug up the strength and patience and, armed with *The Baby Book*, we brought Jordan into our bed. Though his night waking continued, he was much quicker to settle, and a kind of calm overcame our house at bedtime.

Jordan started eating solids at seven months and, despite his apparent suffering, he continued to thrive. He grew and developed alarmingly quickly and conquered each new obstacle easily, only to search for a new challenge. He is (mentally and physically) very strong and healthy. It was not easy but we persevered and with the support of a select few friends with the same beliefs, we lived with the shaky confidence that someday we would reap the rewards of our efforts.

Well, as I gaze adoringly at my energetic, confident toddler, I know that those rewards are coming back to us tenfold. He is still high-need in some ways, but he sleeps through the night, has few fears, is very determined, will try anything, is outgoing and friendly, and attracts people like magnets because of his sparkling personality.

As they say, there are two lasting things you can give your child – roots and wings. I live with the hope that these few demanding and wonderful years have built strong roots from which Jordan can grow. And as we continue to nurture him with unconditional love, we pray that his wings will grow big and strong along with his confidence to use them.

why doesn't this baby sleep?

Now that I have had three children, I reflect a lot on why my first two (especially the first) were high-need.

My husband has a saying that all babies are high-need, some just more than others. He says this because of how we came to realize just how much a baby needs his mother and his parents' time. When our first son, Joe, was born, we didn't have much experience with babies, and most of what we knew came from watching our friends with their baby and from books and magazines. What an awakening (literally and figuratively) we had with Joe! He didn't sleep very much at all, and that became a big issue. I'd ask everyone, "Why doesn't this baby sleep?" He also cried a lot and seemed colicky. As soon as he would fall asleep and I would try to lay him down, he would awaken and cry. Many times I was in tears, too, feeling exhausted and disappointed. Joe always cried in situations where there was a large group of people; I was very apprehensive about taking him to family get-togethers or parties. Joe would cry so hard when I changed his nappy that he would hold his breath and practically turn blue! Yet Joe was as intensely happy as he was fussy. While he fought against sleep, I feel it was his love of and zest for life that kept him awake so much.

I'm sorry that Joe had to go through all that, but I feel in some ways it was what led me to question much of the accepted, well-meaning, and erroneous advice (even medical advice) about babies and children. Once I did that and started to educate myself, I felt better as a mother. I felt it was okay to hold him all the time and natural for me to feel anxious about leaving him. I learned to trust my instincts, and once I could do that, I could deal with my intense little baby.

Having a supportive husband made all the difference in the world, too. Neither of us ever felt comfortable "just letting the baby cry", as we were so often advised to do. We held Joe a lot (almost constantly), even when he was asleep. Unfortunately, I never got used to slings or carriers, so my husband's share in the holding was essential.

How is Joe now? At four years old, he is a great joy to us. He is outgoing and secure, bright and friendly. He is also robust, which is the best adjective I can think of to describe him. He has always been very energetic and intense and he still is. To this day, if he cries, he cries LOUD. He puts his all into whatever he does. He seems very mature and responsible for his age too.

I'm happy to say that now I know! I know a baby needs to be in arms. That is natural.

Anything else is desensitizing. I know it makes sense to sleep near your breast-feeding baby. A mother gets so much more rest this way. I know that it's okay to feel attached to my baby and to trust my instincts. I guess I knew all along. I wish I had been more truly educated and confident when Joe was first born. Sometimes I wish I could do it all over again (or do I?). The most important point I'd like to make is that if you meet the needs of a baby and youngster in the beginning, he will be much more secure and happy, and the mother-child relationship will be more positive later on. I feel I have proof of this in my two high-need young sons. I am glad I devoted myself to them and respected their needs (and I am still doing that) because I can already see what a difference it has made.

day-care nightmare

My son is a bonafide high-need baby, who, at the tender age of eleven months, had already been "expelled" from three day cares! It has been an emotional roller coaster to deal with him, yet I can truly say that I feel closer to him than I did to my first two children, whom I breast-fed but did not practise attachment parenting with.

Seth breast-fed heartily on the delivery table for thirty minutes after birth. However, we rapidly became a rather unhappy feeding couple as he quickly became colicky. The next night in the hospital, both he and I were up the entire night while he cried and I tried to comfort him. (I could recognize the telltale colicky signs from my other two boys' experiences.) The next morning I mentioned to the nurse that he had been crying all night and that neither one of us had slept much. To my surprise, she became quite irate and insisted that I should have left him in the nursery so that I could sleep. Her exact words were "You get them for eighteen years, we only do for one or two nights." I firmly replied that I wanted him with me, and that he should have his own mother to comfort him when he felt bad. I also think that she was somewhat disconcerted by the obvious fact that he had been with me in my bed, and not in the cot at all.

I took Seth home, where he cried night and day. I was truly beside myself. I even tried (unsuccessfully) to open up a day care in my home rather than go back to work (I'm a respiratory therapist) so that I could be with him. I couldn't imagine anyone taking care of, let alone nurturing, my precious baby who needed so much attention. He took only a couple of fifteen-minute naps a day, most often while I held him. Unfortunately, he hated the sling at first. I started to notice a pattern with his behaviour – that it was worse whenever I drank milk. So we went to the local allergist (who is also a paediatrician), who skin-tested Seth and found him to be severely allergic to cow's milk and, less so, wheat and eggs. I was rather devastated at the news, but I was determined not to give up breast-feeding. The health-food store was a godsend, also the La Leche League group. They were very helpful in getting me to think of all that I could eat, rather than all that I couldn't. Seth also had severe eczema.

I wish that I could say that these changes affected him 100 per cent. They didn't, although he was definitely better. However, he still insisted on being held nearly all the time, and at night the only way that he would sleep was nestled next to me. (He still sleeps with me at the age of fifteen months, and still craves closeness.)

Day care has been a nightmare. The first one, which he and I both liked, closed, and three others since have kicked him out. I felt horrible anyway, leaving my precious baby with a harried caregiver who obviously did not like him. When I picked him up he would sometimes be crying, and they would report that they had had to hold him nearly all day. So I finally put an ad in the paper stating very clearly what I wanted, adding that this person must have a great deal of love, and be able to give a large amount of attention to a high-need baby. I also decided to pay extra, which totally ate up the last raise that I received, but I figured that my baby was my most precious commodity. Anyway, it worked. A wonderful woman who has three boys of her own called, and Seth now goes to her house and loves it there. He still screams when I leave (actually, he cries even at home when I leave the room), but I can hear him quieting even as I get into the car. And, best of all, she truly likes him and has a very nurturing personality. I would encourage anyone else who is not entirely happy with their day care to advertise, because there are many differences among caregivers.

Seth is a very devoted breast-feeder, even now. When I pick him up from day care, he dissolves into tears if I don't feed him right away. He refused any solids until he was over ten months, and I was able to pump enough to nourish him. I have decided to let him wean himself, and faced with his strong attachment to me, I wonder if we won't have a few more years of breast-feeding pleasure.

When I'm at work, I don't bring up the subject of breast-feeding anymore. There are countless people who thought that I was off my rocker for avoiding all of those foods. (I was able to eat wheat and eggs after a couple of months, but I still must avoid all milk products.) They also make no secret of the fact that they don't pick up their babies every time they cry. Several people couldn't understand why I pumped for so long either (until he was thirteen months, and I still would be if not for their looks). However, I still pump when I get home and on days off. I've grown accustomed to being a radical (in others' eyes), and to having people think that my baby is a spoiled brat. I feel that I know what is best for him, and luckily I have the support that I need though La Leche League and your books.

It would be unfair not to include how having a high-need baby affects the rest of the family. My boys, aged nine and eleven, were unprepared for the changes that came over us; however, they have become expert nurturers and, I feel, they will become wonderful fathers. At first I heard comments from them relating to breast-feeding such as "gross", and "You're actually going to pump?" However, they are big breast-feeding advocates now, and they make no secret of the fact that they feel sorry for formula-fed babies.

As for Seth's frequent crying and demanding personality, that has been difficult. I am able to stretch only so far, and I don't feel as if I've given my other boys the attention that they deserve. I've consoled myself by thinking that people used to have large families and therefore would naturally not have a lot of time for the older children. Anyway, things are improving, ever so gradually. Just a couple of nights ago Seth started falling asleep before me (previous to this he would fight sleep and succumb only if I fell asleep too; not even pretending to sleep would work).

This has enabled me to spend a little one-on-one time with the older two. I must say that they haven't any malice toward him; indeed, they both love him dearly.

I probably haven't done justice to how demanding my baby is. Until a month or two ago I had to hold him the entire time while I grocery shopped, otherwise he would scream and bother everyone. I never get to shower alone, as he takes only a minuscule nap each day, and he cries miserably unless he is in the shower with me. Until he started walking he wanted to be carried constantly, and to feed very frequently. There are still times that he will want to "marathon nurse". I still carry him most of the time when we go to the shopping centre. (I'm glad that I have a pushchair, although it's used for purchases, definitely not for him!) He has a terrible temper, and he screams very loudly if he does not get what he wants. I used to try to accommodate him in an attempt to hold the peace, until I realized that I'm not doing him any favours by giving in all the time. Also, he rarely plays by himself with his toys; he seems to require someone to interact with him all the time.

Yes, it gets very wearing, and no, I do not have infinite patience. However, and this may sound very egocentric, I have thanked God several times for giving this baby to me rather than to someone who would just give up on him and let him cry it out. What helps me is the fact that I have two older sons, so I realize that this too shall pass. Day by day it seems hard, but I know that there is a light at the end of the tunnel, and that someday our good relationship will be all of the payment that I need.

i snuggled with my premmie in bed

My third child, Jillian, was born at twenty-eight weeks due to premature rupture of the membranes and a subsequent uterine infection from E. coli bacteria. She weighed two pounds, six ounces. She had to remain in the hospital, forty-two miles from our home, for seven weeks. Despite her small size, she was strong and healthy, and her stay in the Special Care Baby Unit was medically uneventful. She had no complications, very little oxygen support, and she made steady progress until I was able to bring her home five weeks before her due date. And while I feel immensely grateful for the miracle of her life and for the excellent medical care she received, I regret that her start in life was so different from the peaceful entry and transition I believe babies need. She is a high-need infant, and I don't know if it is caused by her prematurity, her experience in the SCBU, a genetic predisposition, or a combination of these things.

I began pumping my breasts the day Jillian was born, and she has grown to thirteen pounds in these nine months on my milk. It was tricky, but we made the transition to complete breast-feeding two months after her homecoming. It was stressful because feedings sometimes included using a supplement, giving a bottle, then pumping. This was a day-and-night routine for me.

We first saw evidence of her high-need personality when she would be awake for twelve hours straight during the night. There was very little sleep for me then, having two other children to care for. Even if my husband was up to help feed her, I still had to be up to pump! But I believe our ultimate success at breast-feeding was thanks to my relentless pumping, every two hours for four months.

Anyway, there came a point when exhaustion overwhelmed me. Our other children had slept with us as babies, but, to be honest, I was afraid to put this tiny baby (three pounds, thirteen ounces when she came home!) in bed with me. I feared my breast would smother her. Her nose was the size of the tip of my pinkie! But on one fateful night, after weeks of walking the floor with a crying baby, I snuggled her in bed with me. I decided one night without bottles or pumping would be okay. We were there for seven hours. It was heaven! From then on we went to bed together, and we slept! She would feed frequently during the night, but she never cried. This was also the beginning of our transition to total breast-feeding.

I was amazed at her need for physical closeness to me, despite the fact that she'd spent most of her life alone in an incubator. I embraced this need with joy! Those primal instincts are not easily squelched. And I began to see her high-need personality as a positive sign.

Looking on the bright side, high-need babies have finely tuned survival instincts.

Jillian remains very high-need, and, while I don't know what the future holds, I have developed some strategies that work well in our family.

Besides sleeping with us at night, Jillian sleeps well only in my arms. I gave up trying to move her into the cot for a nap months ago. She will sometimes sleep for a while in her infant carrier in the den or wherever family activity is going on.

I also use my sling a lot. I've learned to do nearly everything but take a shower while wearing Jillian in the sling. I've found that the stimulation of all the activity in the "outer world" (shopping centres, family gatherings, etc.) upsets her if she's in the buggy, but not so much if she's in the sling. She seems most disturbed by strange voices, as she constantly searches for their source. If she's particularly agitated, a warm bath works wonders for her. She's a very clean baby!

The hard part about having a high-need baby is that she requires so much energy, and there is a lot of time involved in meeting her needs. Over the past months it's been hard to give my other children the time and attention they need. Jillian's integration into the family has not gone as smoothly as I imagined it would with a third child.

But the positive side of her neediness is that it's helped to make up for the time we were separated. People often comment, "Oh, your baby is so alert!" I laugh to myself and think they have no idea what an "alert" baby she is!

a screaming bundle of unhappiness

When I was pregnant, I used to sit in the newborn nursery where I worked as a Registered Nurse at night and snuggle the babies. I'd lay them across my chest and feel the warmth of their soft, furry heads on my neck, and think about the not-too-distant future when I would have my own warm bundle to snuggle with. When Mattea was born, she hated to snuggle like that. She screamed from the moment her skin hit air and didn't stop. I knew I was in real trouble when one of my co-workers said, "I'm certainly glad she's going home with you and not with me!"

The first few weeks postpartum were a nightmare – worse than anything I could have imagined. I had never even considered the possibility that I might have a screamer. Not only did she want to feed constantly, but when she wasn't feeding she was screaming. Not a cry, but a high-pitched, painful, ear-piercing scream. She almost never slept. Those first few weeks she averaged four hours of sleep per twenty-four-hour day, and not all four hours were at once. What's more, she slept only if she was being held. My nights were spent sitting in bed, feeding and then trying to sneak her back to her Moses basket beside the bed, only to wake her up with the slightest movement. So she'd scream, I'd cry, we'd feed some more, and on and on, all night long.

My husband was caught completely off guard by this screaming bundle of unhappiness and withdrew into his own world. We'd go for days without a kind word – or any word – being said. I fell deeper and deeper into an angry depression. I told a friend that if someone came to the door with a puppy, I would gladly trade. She laughed, but I wasn't joking. The person who was planning on baby-sitting when I went back to work was visibly relieved when I told her I wasn't going to take the new job I had so looked forward to. I could almost identify with the woman on a talk show who had put her crying baby in the freezer to get some peace. But mostly I thought about driving off a cliff or just disappearing and never coming back. I have never felt so frightened or hopelessly alone as I did after one week with that screaming baby.

When Mattea was two weeks old, I discovered she had a hernia. I was so ashamed to admit it at the time, but I was actually excited to see it! It meant that maybe something really was wrong with this baby – something that could be fixed. It gave me hope that I might actually have a future with this baby.

We spent the next two weeks counting down to the day of her surgery. Christmas was a blur. Nothing mattered except the possible light that was at the end of this miserable tunnel of existence for my husband, our baby, and me.

After the surgery, she still cried a lot, fed a lot, and slept very little, but the high-pitched, painful screaming was less. I was still exhausted and unhappy, but I had felt a pang of fear when she went into surgery that surprised me and made me feel better. It meant that I didn't hate her like I thought I did. I really did want her to be okay.

We struggled with her unhappiness and our horrible feelings of inadequacy for several months until a friend gave me the name of a La Leche League leader. I desperately needed some support, so I called her, even though she was almost four hundred miles away and I had never met her. She reinforced my commitment to continue breast-feeding when all my "support people" had tried to get me to quit with the usual "you're starving her", "your milk is bad" arguments and I had even sneaked her formula once or twice. I still had enough wits about me to know she wasn't starving and that she was physically healthy, but she was still so unhappy. Jackie (the LLL leader) sent me books on breast-feeding, high-need babies, nighttime parenting, and so on, and I devoured them as fast as I could. Mattea wouldn't feed if I read or watched TV. I had to be paying attention to her or she'd cry. But she sometimes would fall asleep at my breast, and then I would read for as long as she slept. The more I read, the better I felt. The books gave me permission to do what I had wanted to do in the first place but felt wasn't "allowed". I stopped trying to sneak her into a cot, a process that usually took several hours and usually failed, and fed her to sleep in our bed. She stayed there and slept a lot more, and so did I. I continued to feed her on demand, which was a lot, but stopped feeling guilty about it. Either my husband or I carried her everywhere. A carrier or backpack became part of our everyday attire. When I went back to work (part-time nights) she slept on my husband in the recliner we bought because she wouldn't sleep in the bed without me.

By the time she was six months old, she was sleeping two to three hours at a time at night, so I got six to eight hours of sleep. Granted, it was interrupted sleep, but it was so much better than it had been. Then we took her to her six-month check-up. I felt good about how far we had come. We were totally in love with her by now. When our doctor said, "There is absolutely no reason a six-month-old baby shouldn't sleep through the night", I was devastated. But by the time we'd made the forty-mile-drive home, I was angry. At that point, we made the decision to leave the medical advice up to the doctor but the parenting advice to our hearts and to the wealth of information and guidance available from LLL.

Mattea is two and a half now. She still needs almost constant attention. She can't sit still or play well by herself like her friends do, but she is a happy and loving child. She is friendly, outgoing, and full of fun. She has been known to walk up to a total stranger who looks sad and try to make them feel better. She certainly still has a rebellious streak, but I wouldn't trade her for anything, not even a puppy! I pray that if we have another child it won't be like she was. But if it is, now we could handle it. We've become wiser and stronger because of her and the help we got from LLL. And if someday we have a quiet, "normal", happy baby, we'll consider ourselves doubly blessed and enjoy it.

The worst part about having a high-need, high-stress baby was the lack of support and understanding from family, friends, and medical professionals. The silver lining to that cloud was discovering a loving way of parenting that we would otherwise never have sought out.

sleepless in canada

Kelly rocketed into the world at 6:42pm on Thursday, March 3, 1994. Although she was much smaller than we had expected at 6 pounds 13 ounces, she was a strong and healthy little soul. She nursed with great enthusiasm in the delivery room shortly after birth, and remained with me constantly during our brief hospital stay. Shortly after her arrival home, Kelly developed jaundice, and spent the next ten days sleeping almost constantly. She was awake only long enough to feed, and even then I had to awaken her for several feedings each day. My husband, Bruce, and I remember how worried we were about our little jaundiced baby and laugh … those first ten days were the only time since Kelly's birth that I have had more than four hour's sleep per twenty-four-hour period!

Once the jaundice had cleared up, we quickly became aware that we were the proud parents of a truly extraordinary baby. Kelly was incredibly alert for so young a child and went for exceptional lengths of time between sleep periods. She was avidly interested in her surroundings and decided very early on that she wanted to be in the middle of everything that I was doing. Before long, I had completely given up any hope of ever putting our child down, as she began to cry the instant that she was away from me. I became intimate friends with a second-hand carrier and a pink sling that a La Leche League associate had made for me, and learned to do practically everything with a baby in arms. The combination of very frequent feeding and being "worn" usually kept Kelly fairly content, although for the first three or four months, she would have several "fussy" periods a day when she demanded more of me. During those times, we would go for walks (again with Kelly being "worn"; we never bought a pushchair, as it seemed like a wasted investment for our special kind of baby!), vacuum together, and, if all else failed, turn on reggae music and bop 'til we dropped! By this time in Kelly's life, I had literally devoured *The Fussy Baby* and was surprised when your suggestion of using classical music to soothe a baby didn't work. Both Bruce and I love Mozart, Vivaldi, Bach, and Chopin, but Kelly hated them! If the music didn't have a driving reggae beat, Kelly wanted no part of it. Needless to say, Bob Marley and the Wailers got a lot of airtime in our house!

These early months passed for me in a blur of constant sleep deprivation. Bruce was a fantastic help with the housework, meal preparation, and moral support, but he was relatively inexperienced with babies, and Kelly seemed to prefer my constant company anyway. We discovered very early on that our little angel was just not a "cot baby": if I couldn't fit in it, Kelly didn't want to sleep in it. Since Bruce holds a very demanding job, I didn't want to have him awakened repeatedly during the night, so I elected to sleep with Kelly in a twin bed in her room. I use the term "sleep" loosely, of course, as I spent most of the night walking the floors with Kelly in my arms. The moment I was still, she would begin to howl. After six months of sleeping in separate quarters, I tossed aside my lofty ambitions to ensure Bruce a good night's sleep. Kelly and I moved into the queen-size bed with Daddy, and we have remained together as a family unit ever since. This move, however, didn't improve our baby's sleeping patterns. Sleep, or the lack thereof, was rapidly becoming the most difficult problem I would face with our high-need baby.

That being said, I did manage to enjoy our daughter very much during this time. She was so incredibly different from other babies of the same age. She was demanding, exhausting, inconsistent, and frustrating, but she had a real spark to her that other children lacked. Kelly was very perceptive right from the word "go", and her responses to me were priceless. Even when she was only a few months old, she would laugh with great enthusiasm if I did something funny, and she would study my every action with intense interest. Her tremendous intelligence radiated from her pretty little face. I used to joke with my mother that Kelly would learn everything I know by the time she was a year old!

Kelly's seventh month was the hardest month for me, although Kelly was much more alert and mobile by this time. For some unknown reason, Kelly decided that she needed even less sleep then, and for about eight weeks she slept for less than seven hours over a twenty-four-hour period and for never more than an hour at a time. I was exhausted, especially since Kelly was still adamant that she wanted to be carried almost constantly (I had begun using a baby backpack by this time, which really helped to distribute her weight). I couldn't figure out what was causing her sleeplessness. I knew that it was nothing she'd eaten, for she didn't start solid foods in earnest until she was almost thirteen months old and was doing very well on breast milk alone. I didn't think that my diet was the problem, as I ate well-balanced meals, didn't smoke or consume alcohol, and had stopped eating or drinking anything that contained caffeine. To this day, Kelly sleeps very little, and I am at a loss to work it out. Perhaps she is just one of those incredible people that needs very little sleep in order to function. [Author's comment: this baby could be sensitive to something in mother's breast milk.]

Strangely enough, our turning point came, not through any dramatic change in Kelly's behaviour, but through a change in my attitude. For months I had been dragging myself around saying, "I'm tired, I'm irritable, and I can't wait until my little girl sleeps through the night." All of a sudden, it dawned on me that I had been surviving in spite of myself, and had kept relatively healthy without the extra sleep that I had been craving. I began to accept that sleeping through the night was just not going to be a realistic goal for Kelly, and my new attitude became, "So, my little girl isn't much of a sleeper … she's thriving, and I'm not doing too badly myself. Why not stop worrying about sleep and get down to the serious business of enjoying my baby?" As soon as I acknowledged that my attitude was largely affecting how lousy I felt, I began to feel better. I still wake up in the morning thinking, "Why can't I have just another half hour's sleep?" but after five minutes of denial, I shake off the blues and get on with the day. Kelly is such a wonderful child, and she is truly a pleasure to wake up to.

The months have all flown by so rapidly, and already I find myself parenting a frenetically active sixteen-month-old. My toddler is every bit as high-need as she was as a baby, but we have such a deep understanding of each other that this rarely poses much of a problem anymore. She is still very demanding, very tiring, and extremely sensitive to over-stimulation or sudden changes to her environment, but to me, she is an absolute delight to parent. Kelly is so bright and inquisitive. Her intense moods are actually becoming a source of encouragement to me, as they may serve her well in later life. In my mind, passionate people are fascinating, creative individuals, who are not afraid to pursue their dreams. Kelly's avid curiosity about the world around her has caused her to be knowledgeable beyond her years. Bruce and I talk to her as most people talk to their three- and four-year-olds. Her speech is still limited, of course, but her comprehension is incredible. High-need babies are a heck of a challenge, but the rewards are tremendous!

career derailed

Danielle, our first child, had really allowed me to continue life as I had lived it before having children. She slept through the night (ten to twelve hours straight) from the age of two weeks, never had nappy rash, and never showed signs of teething until we saw teeth! I returned to work part-time when she was four weeks old and combined that with continuing graduate work and teaching/research when she was a mere nine months! She smiled a lot, loved anyone and everyone, was content with the breast, the bottle, and with or without a dummy. She was very social, and my husband and I spent our first night at a motel without her when she was only two months old.

I just couldn't understand what the big deal was about parenting! Why were those other parents complaining? You just have to do it right, I thought. Set the limits; don't let the children run your life or your household! Keep your own life and your relationship with your husband top priority! It seemed to me that people just let their kids run their lives and that was the problem. Well, thankfully, we hadn't done that! I was never going to have children sleeping in my bed!

And then came Rachael. We had agreed on her name three months before she was even conceived. Good thing, too, as there were many things to come upon which we could not easily agree. The timing of Danielle's and then Rachael's conception was perfectly planned so their births would coincide with my brief respite before returning to my over-achieving teaching schedule! My husband, Larry, had done the majority of Danielle's care while I counselled, taught, did research, and continued university. I thought everything would be just as smooth following Rachael's arrival.

Rachael fed hungrily and eagerly immediately upon her birth and was not happy to be taken away to be examined. I hadn't even been able to get Danielle to feed until she was several hours old! During our brief hospital stay, Rachael screamed whenever she was away, however briefly, from my physical presence. So, needing rest, I had her sleep with me and she fed non-stop. My milk came in like a waterfall twenty-four hours after her birth and she kept the supply coming with her seemingly endless desire to feed.

I enjoyed her closeness and her preference for me over others, though I had a difficult time explaining to my almost one-and-a-half-year-old why Rachael was *always* on my lap. I quickly learned to hold the two of them together and they didn't seem to mind sharing me. I thought the absolute lack of time for myself would be temporary, and it was, though not as temporary as I was thinking then.

Caring for two was harder than caring for one had been, so I allowed Rachael to sleep with Larry and me at night, just so I could get some rest. During the day the girls and I napped altogether in my bed or on the double mattress and on the floor in the girls' room. I kept thinking I was starting a bad habit, but it was so cosy … and, besides, it seemed better than letting Rachael cry herself to sleep. I had never had to do that with Danielle and I felt sure I would never have to with Rachael either. She would change soon, I thought, and then she'd start sleeping in the cot. Such a nice cot, too, matching the dresser and changing table. I had a lovely mental image (more a fantasy!) of Rachael sleeping peacefully there, the whole night through. I was sure it wouldn't be long. But, for now, I would just try to take care of her needs.

Rachael's around-the-clock feeding and wanting to be held by me did not let up one iota by the time she was four weeks old. A couple with whom I had been working in therapy were very eager for me to return to sessions with them, and frankly, I felt a little time out of the house would feel nice. Truthfully, though, I wasn't sure how it was going to work out, as I had yet to use the bathroom without my two companions, one of whom cried the entire minute and a half that it took!

Nevertheless, I made an appointment with my clients, and Larry set his schedule so that he would be available to care for the kids. He had had no practice with Rachael, though, as she would not let anyone hold her without screaming in what we called her "falsetto" voice. Really, a scream with a shrill "vibrato" would be a better description. In any case, it was very clear when she was unhappy. Larry and I, in a good moment, would laugh, and comment that she certainly was a good communicator, having no trouble at all making her feelings known.

Two or three weeks in a row I attempted that one appointment, but by the time I arrived at the office (twenty minutes from home), Larry would already be on the phone, frantically begging me to come home. I could hear Rachael screaming in the background. And Danielle, naturally a very content child, would become very upset at these times, knowing Daddy did not have whatever it was that Rachael was needing, however hard he tried.

Finally, my clients suggested I bring Rachael with me! They were expecting their first child and felt it would be good practice for them to be exposed to such a young infant. I thought the idea of a therapist bringing her newborn with her to counselling sessions was hilarious, but we tried it. For several sessions, Rachael came along with me as I tried to play professional, meanwhile having to leave the office periodically to soothe her, eventually learning to feed her under a shawl while I talked with my clients.

This whole situation left me feeling very uneasy. I felt I was not meeting the needs of my clients or my baby and it was making me a nervous wreck! I finally told my clients that I would have to stop for a "few weeks" until Rachael was able to stay home with my husband. I was sure it wouldn't be long; I had just been rushing things. I was beginning to see that Rachael was different than Danielle had been. And, since I wasn't willing (nor was my husband!) to have her just "deal with" my being gone, I decided to try to go with the flow.

By September, Rachael was four months old and I had to notify the university that I would not be able to teach that term. Besides teaching and preparation time, I knew the forty-five-minute drive would make the time away impossible. I felt much like a prisoner by this time, as Rachael hated being in the car. I had never heard of such a thing! A baby who didn't like being in the car?! Isn't a ride in the car supposed to be the cure for any fussy baby? Well, not this one! Our church was only a ten-minute drive from our home, but we had to pull over at least once to feed and soothe her and survive the rest of the ride with her upset. Between that and spending the entire service in the nursery with Rachael week after week, we finally quit going.

On the positive side, I was really enjoying the closeness I felt to my daughters. It was nice to be able to spend time with them, not having to rush through anything. Actually, a completely open schedule was the only way I could survive. The girls and I just kept plodding along, one day running into the next, no deadlines, just napping together, bathing together, meeting the basic needs of the household in an on-again, off-again sort of way. I did receive remarks from others about how I was spoiling Rachael and I remembered having been on the other side!

On one occasion when she was four weeks old, I made an attempt to go out with Rachael, even though it meant a ride in the car, which, as I said, made her scream non-stop. I was determined to see my husband play baseball at least once, and the season was almost over. It was only a twenty-minute drive to the ball field and I had already pulled over three or four times to soothe her. So, I reached over and rubbed her tummy and kept explaining to her that we were almost there.

Rachael did not stop crying, and when we made it to the field, I parked the car and took her out of the car seat to comfort her. Rachael continued to cry hysterically for forty minutes no matter what I did. She wouldn't even feed! This was so upsetting to me that I started crying, finally. Eventually, Rachael "passed out" from the sheer exhaustion of crying.

For the next couple of days, Rachael cried a little when she slept, as if she was having bad dreams, remembering the experience. I felt so much regret over having let her cry and worried that she might have emotional damage from it! Friends told me I was overreacting and said she really had me trained! Although I wasn't successful reasoning with them, all I could do was listen to my instincts and learn to live peacefully with my daughter. I just kept reminding myself that Rachael had only one mother and that she was counting on me to understand her and be there for her.

My husband is still wondering when things are going to return to "normal". He is very supportive, accepting my interpretation of the situation and giving me room to do what I think is best for our children. We now occasionally go out together and enjoy the times the sitter takes the girls for a walk for a half hour or so!

The best news of all is that Rachael is a very expressive and loving one-year-old! She kisses everyone and exudes joy to everyone around her. She walks around smiling, laughing, and squealing with delight and is very giving and sharing and comforting with other children.

Through these past fourteen months I have really come to enjoy my children, and it has been nice to be home full-time. I have, at times, felt completely overwhelmed with the needs of the girls, and I still occasionally go without brushing my hair for a couple days, but I know this time will pass all too quickly. I feel good knowing that I have "done right by" my children and I look forward to any siblings they may have!

he's a hard-to-love baby

I came home from my nine-day stay in the hospital (due to a kidney infection) post C-section desperately weak, with two children to care for. Somehow, with my husband's help, I made it. I was on antibiotics and painkillers for several more weeks, nursing Jacob constantly. If he was not feeding, he was crying, and he would sleep only twenty minutes at a stretch (at the most) during the day and about two hours at a time at night. Even after I started feeling better, he would calm only for a few seconds while being carried, and then wail again. So I would feed him again or change his nappy.

After about three months he developed patches of eczema, and he constantly had dirty nappies. When he was a newborn, I never changed just a wet nappy. I would change about twenty dirty nappies a day! And imagine that I'm doing this with a less-than-two-year-old also in the house! Because Jacob was so chronically irritated, I began to suspect that he was reacting to something in my diet.

I began cutting out more and more items, and finally worked myself down to a very basic diet. His eczema improved, his bowels were not entirely in an uproar, and he didn't cry quite all the time. I had also taken him to a paediatric allergist just to make sure that I wasn't overlooking some rare problem.

Throughout this, however, he was growing and gaining weight. He was always pleasingly plump and never looked like a chronically fussy baby. Soon he started to do all of the normal developmental things, and as my daughter had begun eating solids right around six months, I began trying him on a few very safe home-prepared items. Nothing doing. He had no desire to eat!

But he fed! So I stayed on my diet. And he fed. And he fed. And he refused food. He was eleven months, he was twelve months; it was Thanksgiving, it was Christmas. A bit concerned that I was about to test the limits of how long a child could be sustained solely through breast-feeding, I called La Leche League and got in touch with some other mums whose children had had similar desires. All of them assured me that their children had decided sometime around fifteen months to eat. And so did Jacob.

I had begun taking him (and his sister) to a local Montessori school for the parent-child class, and it was about this time (between eleven and fifteen months) that his disposition began to change. As he grew into toddlerhood, the ceaseless crying stopped, the diarrhoea lessened and then disappeared, and he began to enjoy life. Whereas we had once tickled him just to see him smile or hear him laugh (which he had never done spontaneously as an infant), we now found a happy toddler excited to discover the world.

Jacob will turn three in October, and is at the wonderfully moody age where children discover that they are individuals and want to exercise that individuality constantly. He is slowly learning that hitting others discourages them from playing with him; that Mummy loves him even when she is not in sight; that his sister's things are hers and not Jacob's; and so forth. In other words, a very normal child.

I don't know why his infancy was so trying. If there was one thing that got me through everything, it was breast-feeding. Jacob was a very hard-to-love infant, and if I had not breast-fed him, I'm certain that we would not be as close as we are today.

the proof is in the pudding

I should have suspected something was up when I was pregnant. Barney was a very active foetus. We have video of him flipping around inside me (not ultrasound video, a home video; he was that visible). People used to stare at my rumbling abdomen! Barney went through a very traumatic three-day labour and a very medicated and intervention-filled delivery.

He had colic. Oh, boy, did he have colic! All he did was scream, day and night. The onslaught of "let-him-cry-it-out" advice had begun. We didn't know what to do! My heart kept telling me no! He needed comforting, but we were inundated with "helpful" advice. And I certainly didn't want a "family bed". No way! I wasn't one of those hippie, weirdo, yoghurt-weaving women. So Barney cried in a cradle (hand-built by my husband) by our bed. Finally, exhausted, I went to a mum-to-mum meeting at our hospital, and a woman there (now a dear friend) suggested your book *Nighttime Parenting*. I still protested, "I don't want to be a nighttime parent. I want to be a daytime parent – just make him stop!" I caved and bought your book. It literally changed all our lives.

Now I understood that our high-need baby needs high-need parenting, day and night. I kept a journal and I looked back at what our nights were like: Barney would eat forty minutes, burp for twenty minutes, and fuss to sleep for thirty minutes. He'd sleep for thirty minutes and then start all over. This gave me at most thirty minutes of sleep every two hours (if I fell right to sleep!). This went on for the first six weeks. What worked was bringing him to bed. He ate better and slept better, and so did I.

I also had to keep reminding myself that nothing was as important as my baby, everything could wait. In order to take the best care of my baby, I absolutely needed to rest whenever he rested. This "mantra" I said over and over as I looked at the dishes, laundry,

floors. I still do this many days, even now that our high-need angel is ten and a half months old. (In fact, I'm writing this next to him as he sleeps. He sleeps better with me here.)

I always start any project with the intention of being able to drop it. I compliment myself on any progress made ("Well, at least I got the plates picked up" instead of "Can't you at least let me load the dishwasher?") Remembering that my high-need baby needs more and needs it now helps with any frustration I might feel.

Six months ago I would have been hard-pressed to state any positives about having a high-need baby. It was so exhausting. Having a high-need baby is a trial by fire. It forces you to re-evaluate your priorities. (I had planned on going back to work and having a nanny!) I've had people say to me, "If I had a baby like that, I wouldn't have anymore." To that I have to smile, although I wouldn't wish another high-need baby on myself. I have mixed feelings. I worry a regular-need baby would be boring! I feel after Barney, I'm ready for another! He keeps me constantly challenged, constantly burning. I say Barney lives life large. He does everything with gusto, including loving me. When he runs to me and gives me a hug, I know it's genuine. He really needs me and my love. I'm guiding this high-need spirit in positive directions, and I know he'll do great things in life. My husband and I have had some trying times with him, but it has definitely drawn us closer. He has been a true blessing.

Having the confidence to stand up for your high-need baby and his needs is important – confidence to stand up to the "let-him-cry-it-out", "you're spoiling him", "you'll pay for this later", "don't you need to get a baby-sitter?" "He'll be fine" people. It takes confidence to say, "My baby needs me now, no, we can't go to the business dinner." People think you're nuts! A friend of ours says, "The proof is in the pudding." I can already see the proof in Barney. People always comment what a happy baby he is. (A big change from "Boy, he cries a lot. You should give him a break, maybe it's your milk.") Barney started walking at eight and a half months and now he's running! He has confidence to explore new surroundings and new people, knowing he can come to Mum or Dad for reassurance. Barney has always been advanced. He is allowed to develop because his high needs are always met. He doesn't have to waste developmental energy crying or worrying. Yes, the proof is in the pudding.

I wish you could see him in person. He shows the beautiful effects of high-need parenting. He's a great boy. Although I'd pay about a thousand pounds for eight hours of sleep, I wouldn't swap a minute of the time I've spent with him for anything. A high-need baby is a challenge that only the parent of a high-need baby can understand. It is unfortunate that people still think of "good" babies as quiet ones. My high-need baby is not good – he's great!

i would not want her any other way

Having lived for three years feeling as if I have a leech stuck on me, sucking at my energy, needing my lifeblood and love, I feel pretty wiped out. Yet ecstatically happy, too, all at once. I may be worn out, exhausted, and feeling like there is little of me left, but on the other hand, I have a beautiful, intelligent, energetic child who knows more than I could ever imagine and who asks the kind of questions I might expect of a ten-year-old.

I was a young and naive mum who knew only about standard baby care. Caleigh demanded much more of me. She wouldn't give up on me until I came around to her way of thinking. I am so happy that she is as demanding as she is. I am proud of her strength. She carried more strength in her tiny newborn body than many adults do in their grown-up bodies. How anyone can see that as a negative trait I do not understand.

I see many of the traits of high-need children as a sign of strength. They have high needs and they find the means to get them met. Unlike more passive children, they do not give up after a few minutes and stop. They feel a need and they are willing to give their utmost to get it met.

The instantaneous needs of a high-need child can feel demanding and frustrating at times. "I need love now", she seems to be saying. At the same time, she gives her love in an instant, too – with the passion that only a high-need child can feel. High-need children say, "I love you, Mum", just as strongly as "I need you to love me, Mum."

It's important for the parents of a high-need child to keep some perspective. Remember that what exhausts you now will one day put a big smile on your face. Someday this same child will focus her energies on things other than Mum (or

Dad), and she will be able to do many great things.

Sometimes you may wish your child were content to sit and watch television or get involved in some other passive activity so that you could get things done now. But in later years, will you really want her to be so passive? Of course not. You will want her to be active and to participate in life. If you want these things later, you need to learn how to deal with them now. It's not easy. I will never say it is. But it is the best way.

Over time, Caleigh has grown and changed too. She can now be away from me for short periods of time comfortably (usually it's a case of her going out with someone rather than my leaving her behind). In her own way, she is extremely independent and increasingly so. She loves to do things with other people now, like playing on the computer with her uncle Robbie or picking blackberries with Dad and the dog. Separating from Mum is slow, but it does happen.

Remember to take care of yourself and to do what you enjoy. If your child sees you happy and fulfilled, chances are good she will be happy and fulfilled too.

time to move on

We are die-hard fans of attachment parenting – breast-feeding and the family bed have turned our fussy baby into a happy, bright, good-natured, healthy fifteen-month-old. At age forty, I want to start on another baby soon – within the next four months. We've learned to accept our son's frequent night waking and feeding back to sleep, but I can't imagine our sweet babe feeding on and climbing all over my pregnant body, with all its new aches and irritabilities. So, much as I would love to continue feeding, I've had to take inventory of where I'm at in life and move on. Our little guy will gain a great deal more joy and learning from having a sibling than from continuing to breast-feed. I realize that what he really needs now is me, not my breast. He has learned very quickly that his mummy is still there for him. He now goes to sleep peacefully with his hand on "his" breast. My confidence and clearness about my need to wean made it much less a struggle than I'd heard it could be.*

---

*   For more extensive information on weaning, consult *The Baby Book*, by William Sears and Martha Sears (Thorsons, 2005).

index